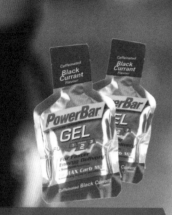

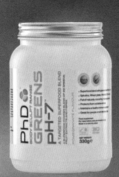

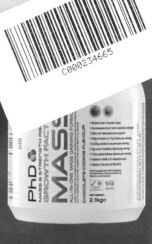

1 ENERGY

It's important that your body has the fuel it needs so you can train at your best. The useable form of energy in your muscles is glycogen, which we get from carbohydrates. Carbs release energy at various speeds and are ranked on what is known as the Glycaemic Index. It's important to get a good mix of low- and high-GI carbohydrates so our bodies have both fast and sustained releases of energy. This, in turn, will provide your energy systems with the fuel for whatever training you have planned.

Powerbar Fast Fuel Gels 24 x 41g

This gel offers a blend of fast-acting carbohydrates, branch chain amino acids (BCAAs) and electrolytes. This will deliver much-needed glycogen to your working muscles. The BCAAs and electrolytes will help to keep your muscles hydrated and balanced, as well as speeding up your recovery.

RRP: £29.99
Monster Price: £28.99
Quickfind: 4405

2 IMMUNE

High training volumes twinned with a busy work or family life can sometimes leave you feeling run-down. It's important to stay on top of your intake of vitamins and minerals through a good diet. This will help you maintain a strong immune system and keep illness at bay. Overtraining can be common problem in endurance sport; by keeping your body fighting fit through your diet you will limit any frustrating setbacks caused by illness.

PhD Nutrition Greens pH -7 330g

This product is ideal for athletes with a high training volume. The superfood blend will help support your immune system, which is especially important for endurance athletes. The vitamin content can help with energy uptake and protection from oxidative stress. We all know how hard it can be to get our five-a-day, so this goes a long way in helping us look after our bodies.

RRP: £34.99
Monster Price: £27.93
Quickfind: 5702

3 RECOVERY

In order to perform well tomorrow, you need to recover well today. Recovery is extremely important in endurance sports because the training volumes are usually very high. For example, if we have a long run on Monday, we may need to recover for a speed session on Wednesday. The best way to do this is to begin refuelling as soon as you finish a session. You then need to maintain this calories intake in the hours after the session. It's important to use both protein and carbohydrates to replenish energy stores and repair any damage to your muscle tissue.

PhD Nutrition Growth Factor Mass 2.1kg

This is a great supplement for recovery or as an energy-boosting supplement when you don't have time for a meal. The five-stage carbohydrate complex means you get fast and sustained-release glycogen replenishment, while the hefty protein content will help with the development and repair of muscle tissue. The products also contains many other ingredients shown to help with both performance and recovery.

RRP: £53.99
Monster Price: £32.29
Quickfind: 5701

EASY NUTRITION FOR RUNNERS: INSIDE

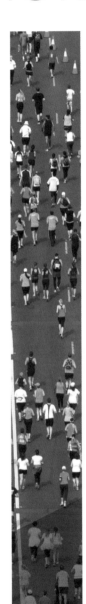

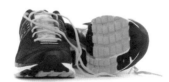

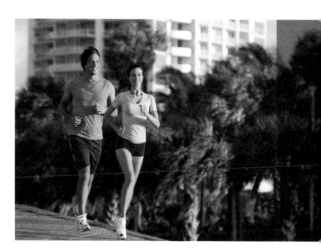

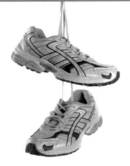

EAT RIGHT, RUN FASTER!

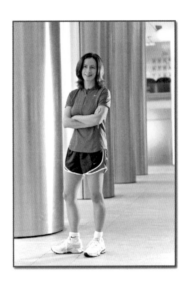

The sheer joy of running can be blighted sometimes by the confusion surrounding nutrition. What should you eat before a run? What's the best food for recovery? What supplements do you need and how often should you take them? Nutrition is, in fact, a minefield, with so many experts offering differing opinions. And if you're someone who, like me, took up running for weight loss, how can you make sure that you're not just cancelling out any benefits by overeating?

This is where our new guide comes in. *Easy Nutrition For Runners*, brought to you by the experts from *Women's Running* and *Men's Running* magazines, is designed to do exactly what the title says: provide you with clear, concise, nutritional advice that won't confuse or bamboozle, in an interesting, informative and appealing way.

This 148-page extensive manual is ideal for all runners, so whether you've just started or you're about to run another marathon, you'll find all the advice you need to help you feel good during your runs and afterwards, when you're recovering.

Good nutrition is too important to overlook, so we want to help you get it right. We start with advice for beginners and go on to tackle nutrition for every race distance – ranging from 5Ks to ultra marathons – so that you can prepare an effective and easy nutrition plan for whatever race distance you're training for. All this, plus tips on recovery, a guide to vitamins and minerals, and even how to cope with runner's trots caused by bad eating habits – we know you'll find *Easy Nutrition For Runners* a guide you'll turn to time and time again.

And if you need motivation to get out and run, visit our websites for advice, training plans and top tips at womensrunninguk.co.uk or mensrunninguk.co.uk.

Christina Macdonald, Editor-in-Chief

women'srunning   **MEN'S Running**

EASY NUTRITION FOR RUNNERS

EDITOR-IN-CHIEF
CHRISTINA MACDONALD
chris.macdonald@wildbunchmedia.co.uk
TEL: 020 8996 5135

CHIEF SUB-EDITOR
CLAIRE CHAMBERLAIN

SUB-EDITORS
**JOHN CARROLL, DANNY COYLE,
JON EDWARDS**

ART EDITOR
JAMES WILKINSON
james.wilkinson@wildbunchmedia.co.uk

ONLINE EDITOR
CARYS MATTHEWS
carys.matthews@wildbunchmedia.co.uk
TEL: 020 8996 5056

COMMERCIAL DIRECTOR
ALLAN PATTISON
allan.pattison@wildbunchmedia.co.uk
TEL: 020 8996 5058

SENIOR ADVERTISING SALES
EXECUTIVE
RHIANNON MATTHEWS
rhiannon.matthews@wildbunchmedia.co.uk
TEL: 020 8996 5090

SALES EXECUTIVE
FIONNUALA COLLINS
f.collins@wildbunchmedia.co.uk
TEL: 020 8996 5104

CIRCULATION MANAGER
HELEN KNIGHT
helen.knight@wildbunchmedia.co.uk

DIRECTOR
NICK TROOP
nick.troop@wildbunchmedia.co.uk

DIRECTOR
KEVIN MCCORMICK
kevin.mccormick@wildbunchmedia.co.uk

CONTRIBUTORS
Christine Bailey, Anita Bean, Kate Blinman, Lynn
Clay, Lyndel Costain, Jill Eckersley, Anne-Marie
Lategan, Jo Scott-Dalgleish

PUBLISHED BY
WILD BUNCH MEDIA LTD
1st Floor, Gable House
18-24 Turnham Green Terrace
London W4 1QP

PRINTED BY
WILLIAM GIBBONS
01902 730011

DISTRIBUTION BY
MARKETFORCE UK LTD
Blue Fin Building
110 Southwark Street
London SE1 0SU
Tel: 020 3148 3300

CHRISTINE BAILEY
Christine is a qualified nutritionist. She is also a professional chef, food and health consultant, and journalist. Christine advises runners, cyclists and sports clubs on nutrition and performance and is the author of *The Intelligent Way To Lose Weight*. Visit www.advancenutrition.com

JO SCOTT-DALGLEISH
Jo is a qualified nutritionist, based in London, who works with runners, cyclists and triathletes to develop a personal nutrition plan that helps improve performance while maintaining good health. She enjoys running, cycling and swimming. Visit her website www.endurancesportsnutritionist.co.uk

JULIET MCGRATTAN
Juliet is a GP, a keen runner and a mother of three. She has been running for four years and has taken part in many races, including the Cross Bay Half Marathon and the Helly Hansen Beauty and the Beast, as part of the *Women's Running* team. This year she ran the Virgin London Marathon for the first time.

ANNE-MARIE LATEGAN
Anne-Marie has a BSc Hons in Human Movement Science & Rehabilitation. She specialises in functional training, body sculpting and orthopaedic rehabilitation. She has run a marathon and several ultra marathons, recently completing a mammoth 120K ultra event.

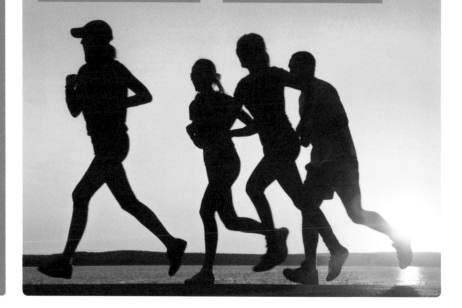

NUTRITION
FOR NEW RUNNERS

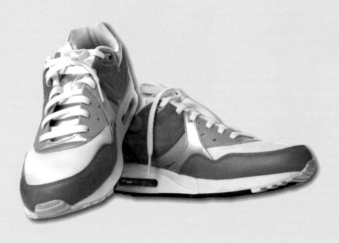

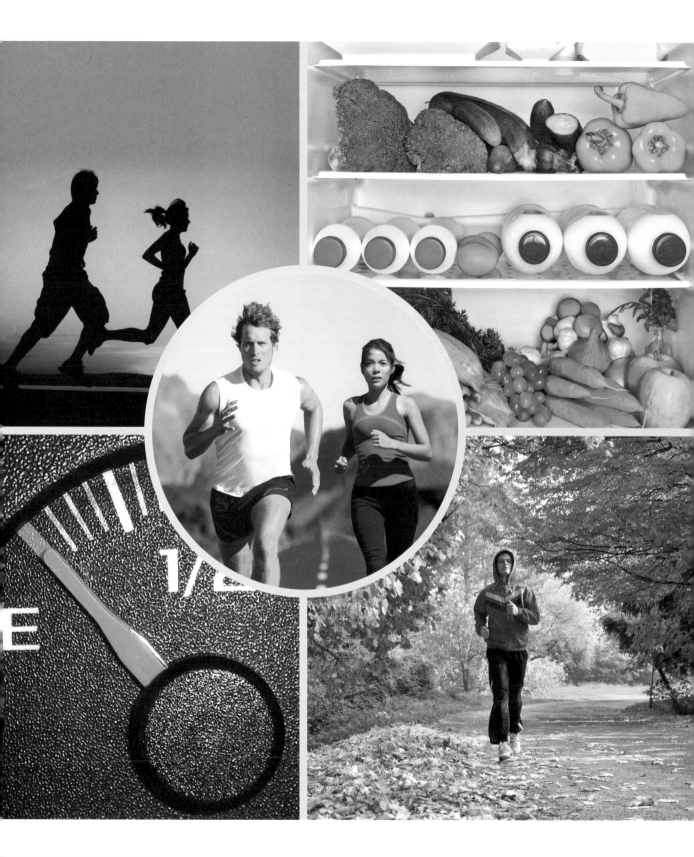

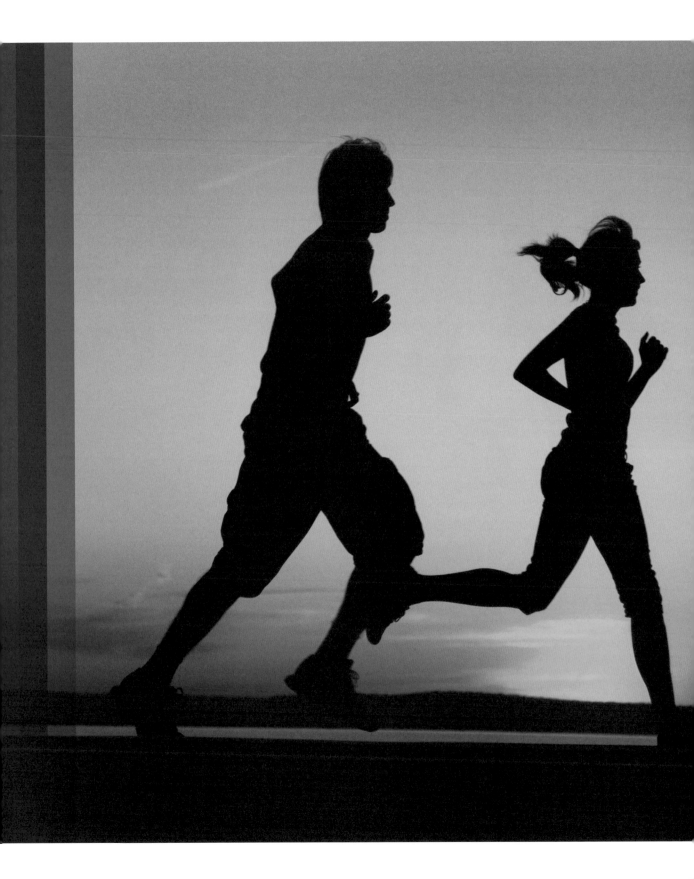

ARE YOU TOTALLY NEW TO RUNNING?

A GOOD DIET IS JUST AS IMPORTANT AS GOOD TRAINING. HERE'S HOW TO GET THE BASICS RIGHT

Whether you decide to run for weight loss, competition, fun or fitness, you need to fuel your body correctly. Get your nutrition right and you will perform better, recover faster and stay injury-free. Here's what you need to know.

ENERGY INTAKE

Even if you are running primarily to lose weight you still need to take in sufficient calories to fuel your body. Body composition-measuring devices at gyms can be used to indicate your basal metabolic rate (how many calories you need to simply fuel your body if you're doing nothing all day except existing). You then need to add on an activity factor to calculate your everyday calorie needs. This can range from 1.2 to 1.7 depending on how active you are – a nutritionist or personal trainer should be able to guide you.

To this figure you add the calories for your running or training sessions (approx. 100 calories per mile or 400-600 calories per hour). Heart rate monitors can tell you exactly how many calories you've burned during a run or exercise session, while gym machines such as treadmills and steppers are also reasonably accurate. But if this seems too complicated, the simplest way to

know if your calorie intake matches your expenditure is to monitor your weight. If you're looking to lose weight aim to keep weight loss to around 2lb per week. Otherwise, a stable weight means you're doing well. (If weight loss is your main aim, see page 114 for the lowdown on foods with hidden calories).

CARBOHYDRATE NEEDS

Carbohydrates are a vital energy source for runners. Glucose derived from carbohydrates is the main type of sugar in the blood and is the body's preferred source of energy. However, we can only store relatively small amounts of glucose in our muscles and liver as glycogen. The more glycogen available, the longer you can keep going at a higher level of performance. Hitting the wall occurs as your carbohydrate reserves run low and your muscles start to use fat as an additional source of energy. As you train more and increase your distance running, your muscles become better at transforming carbs and fat into energy, which means you can run faster for longer.

The amount of carbohydrate-containing foods you eat can influences the amount of glycogen you store. Taking in sufficient carbohydrate before, during and after

exercise provides glucose for energy and helps to speed up recovery and restore glycogen levels, so you're ready for your next training session.

CARBOHYDRATE SOURCES

To keep your energy levels high and avoid energy dips, eat foods that are good sources of carbohydrates, such as wholegrains – from bread, rice, cereal and pasta – as well as fruits and vegetables and some low-fat dairy foods. For most of the time focus on foods with a low glycaemic index – these foods are broken down by the body into glucose at a slower rate, providing more sustained energy. Good examples include porridge oats, wholegrain rice, rye bread, oat cakes, sweet potato and starchy vegetables.

Just before and after training you may need a more rapid energy boost to fuel your training as well as speed up recovery. This is the time to eat quick-releasing, carbohydrate-rich foods such as bananas, cereal bars, dried fruit or fruit smoothies.

GET THE RIGHT FATS

As you increase your running distance, fats become particularly important in your diet as an additional fuel. Medium chain

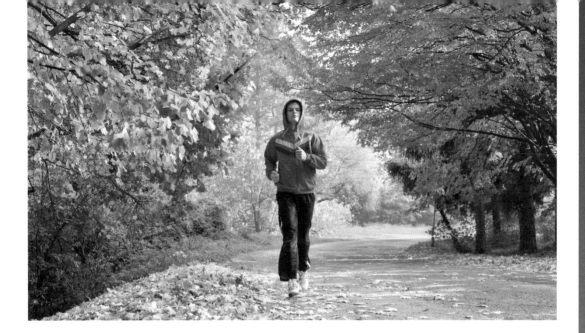

triglycerides, found in coconut oil, for example, can be useful, as they are preferentially burnt by the body and used for energy production. As you increase your mileage try adding a spoonful of coconut oil to your morning smoothie.

All runners need to get the essential fats omega 3 and omega 6 fatty acids from their diet because they cannot be made in the body. Omega 3 fats, in particular, are often low in people's diets yet are hugely important for runners. These fats support tissue growth and repair, promote the production of anti-inflammatory chemicals and reduce the risk of cell damage. They may also aid recovery. To get enough essential fats, try to eat:

• Two or three portions of oily fish (salmon, trout, herring, anchovy, mackerel, sardines) per week. Canned tuna is not a good source of omega 3 fats and fresh tuna can be contaminated by dioxins and mercury so limit consumption. (For more information on fish oils and how they can benefit your running, turn to page 88).

• 1-2tbsp of mixed seeds (eg sesame, pumpkin, sunflower, chia, flaxseed) daily. Eat these as a snack or add them to porridge, smoothies, muesli etc. Alternatively, use 1-2tbsp of hempseed, flaxseed, pumpkin or walnut oil daily.

• Monounsaturated fats, found in olive oil, nuts, seeds and avocados also possess anti-inflammatory properties, so it's a good idea to include some in your diet.

• Use olive oil and coconut oil daily in cooking, dressings or add to dishes.

• Snack on nuts rich in mono-unsaturated fats. Include avocado, olives, nut and seed butters regularly.

PROTEIN

Don't skimp on your protein. Pretty much everything in the body is made of proteins and it's also essential for repair. Running – especially long-distance running – can cause damage to the muscles, joints and other tissues, so ensuring sufficient protein in your diet becomes a priority.

Guidelines for daily protein intake for runners will vary depending on the amount of training you're doing

(see below). An easy way to manage your protein intake is to aim for 15-20g of protein at each meal and to include some protein foods with your snacks too. Good sources of protein include lean meat, fish, eggs, low-fat dairy, beans and pulses, soy, protein powders and, to a lesser extent, green vegetables such as broccoli and spinach. A 100g chicken breast contains around 30g protein, a small pot of cottage cheese (100g) contains 13g, two eggs offer 12g and a small tin of tuna (100g) contains around 24g.

GETTING THE BALANCE RIGHT

As a guide you can base carbohydrate and protein intake on your body weight. The actual amount you need really depends on the amount of exercise you are doing.

Carbohydrate: 5-7 grams per kilogram of body weight per day
Protein: 1.1-1.8g per kg of body weight per day
Fat: 25-30% of total calories

So, for someone who weighs 60kg, this would be around 300-420g carbohydrates and 66-108g protein.

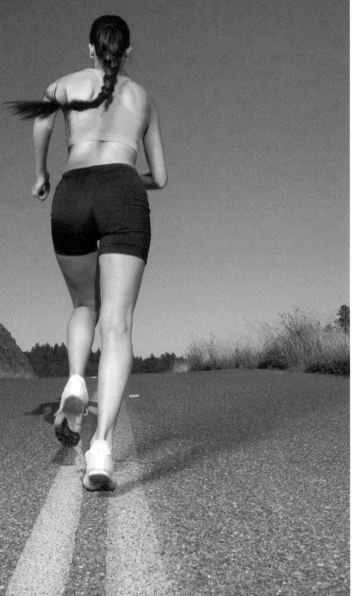

'To avoid energy dips and fatigue you need to replace glycogen stores'

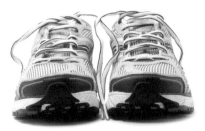

GET THE TIMING RIGHT

It's not just what you eat that makes a difference to your performance but when you eat.

Before a run: For shorter runs (less than an hour), focus on eating some high-carbohydrate foods about 30 minutes before training – this could mean a small, easily digested carbohydrate snack such as a banana, cereal bar or sports drink. For longer runs, eat a larger carbohydrate-based meal about two hours before training to avoid feeling nauseous during the session. This may be a bowl of porridge with some fruit and a handful of nuts and seeds.

During: If you are running for longer than one hour you may need to keep your blood glucose and fluid levels topped up. On average, runners use 60g of carbohydrate per hour so, depending on the length of your run, you may wish to take an isotonic drink or sports gel with you.

After a run: To avoid energy dips and fatigue you need to replace glycogen stores, which requires carbohydrates, but you also need to promote muscle and tissue repair, which requires protein. Without correct refuelling you are less likely to get the most from your training. You may also find your next run feels harder and over time your performance may suffer. You are also more likely to develop muscle soreness and injury. Aim to eat a high-carbohydrate snack with some protein within 30-45 minutes after your run. Good examples include a protein fruit smoothie, cereal bar or some fruit and yogurt. For longer runs eat a larger snack or meal within one hour of finishing. Try an egg sandwich, cottage cheese with a baked potato or chicken with rice and vegetables.

WHY THE WEIGHT GAIN?

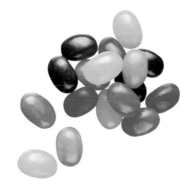

MANY PEOPLE TAKE UP RUNNING TO LOSE WEIGHT, BUT END UP ACTUALLY PUTTING ON A FEW KILOS. IT JUST DOESN'T SEEM FAIR – AND IT DOESN'T HAVE TO HAPPEN

The single biggest mistake made by runners trying to lose weight is thinking they can eat whatever they want, simply because they run. This isn't always the case. It's easy to overestimate the amount of calorie-burning work you do in your run and just as easy to underestimate the calories in the biscuits or ice cream you consume after dinner as a reward. And even if your diet is generally good, you might still be overeating healthy food – all foods contain calories. (Never forget, however, that if you've just started running or if you're increasing your mileage, your weight gain may be the result of extra muscle.)

BALANCING ACT
It's important to think before you eat in order to find the right balance between your running and your diet. As a rule, you will burn between 80 and 100 calories for every ten minutes you run. So a 30-minute run would balance out the calories in one Mars bar. Also, it's common to feel hungry directly after a run. This is because your body's energy stores have been reduced and must be replaced. This is not the time to have that Mars bar. Immediately after your run, you should eat food that's high in protein and has a small amount of carbohydrate. This will help to rebuild your muscles as well as replace the energy in those muscles (muscle glycogen) and in the liver (liver glycogen). Make sure you stock your fridge and food cupboards with healthy foods, so you can easily grab something that's good for you when you come home from a run. Better yet, prepare something before you leave.

TAKE STOCK
Keeping a food and activity diary for a week is a good way to evaluate your habits. On one side of the page write down how long you have run for, how fast and (as accurately as you can) how many calories you have used each day. On the other side, write down what you had for breakfast, lunch, dinner, snacks and everything that you drank, noting how many calories you're consuming. Be honest – some people try to be extra good with their diet when they have to write a food diary, but that will lead to a false reading if you keep up such a diet for only a week. Ensure you write down all your drinks – coffee and tea with sugar, sports drinks, fizzy drinks and fruit juices can add a significant number of calories. At the end of the week you'll have a good idea of whether you're doing enough exercise to justify your calorie intake. Be aware that an average woman needs about 2,000 calories a day while men need 2,500, but this will vary slightly depending on many factors, including age and activity level.

FOOD FOR THOUGHT
Treats are tasty (the clue is in the name), easy to find and often seen as a reward for hard work, but it's worth comparing the calories in a treat with the effort needed to burn them off...

FOOD	MINUTES TO BURN OFF
Mars bar (280 cal)	30
Crisps (192 cal per 40g)	20
Coca-Cola (225 cal per 500ml)	23
Flapjack (300 to 400 cal)	30 to 40
Lucozade Sport (140 cal per 500ml)	14
Medium-sized banana (97 cal)	10

'Immediately after your run, you should eat food that's high in protein and has a small amount of carbohydrate'

DON'T GIVE IN TO CRAVINGS

Sugar cravings are your body's way of telling you that your blood sugar has dropped; it doesn't mean you have to stuff yourself with sugary food. Cravings last for about ten minutes, so the best thing to do is distract yourself for those crucial minutes or go for a healthy option. Keep seeds or nuts in your gym bag to ensure you always have a healthy snack to hand. If you run just before lunch or dinner, try to prepare your meals before you go out. This way you can ensure your food is ready as soon as you get in, which will prevent you from snacking before your meal. Make sure you keep an eye on your portion sizes – use a smaller plate and avoid second helpings. It takes a few minutes for your brain to work out that your stomach is full, so if you still feel hungry, drink some water and wait ten minutes before deciding if you want – or need – to eat more.

WHAT'S THE ALTERNATIVE?

HEALTHY ALTERNATIVES TO UNHEALTHY SUGAR TREATS

» Instead of eating a full packet of M&M's, mix them up with sunflower and pumpkin seeds. This way you get your chocolate treat, but you eat less of it. The sunflower and pumpkin seeds are high in calcium and magnesium, minerals that are important for muscle function and bone strength.

» Add a scoop of protein powder, peanut butter or a seed mix to your smoothie, to increase the protein and mineral content.

» Instead of eating breakfast bars or cereal bars, try a bar that's higher in protein. TREK Protein Bars contain up to 12g of protein and are a good alternative to sugary bars.

HUNGER GAMES

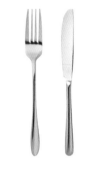

WHAT IF RUNNING DENTS YOUR APPETITE? AND WHAT HAPPENS IF YOU DON'T REFUEL PROPERLY AFTER A RUN?

Most runners know they need to eat a combination of healthy carbohydrates and protein soon after a run to kick-start recovery. But what if you don't feel hungry straight away after a run? If you wait too long for your appetite to return after a long run, you will delay recovery. It takes at least 20 to 24 hours of refuelling with carbohydrate-rich foods to replenish your muscle stores fully, so daily workouts can leave you running on low fuel stores. Since the effects of dehydration and muscle glycogen depletion can be cumulative, inadequate refuelling can contribute to overtraining syndrome (when you push your body beyond its capability, resulting in fatigue, injury, a weakened immune system and mood changes).

WHY DO I SOMETIMES LOSE MY APPETITE AFTER A RUN?

A loss of appetite is quite common after intense exercise. It happens in part because running causes the hypothalamus gland (the brain's hunger centre) to release some of the same neurotransmitters that tell you you're full after eating a meal. Hunger is also suppressed when there are high levels of amino acids and fatty acids in the blood, as is the case after exercise, due to the mobilisation of these nutrients to provide energy during running. High-intensity running increases plasma amino acid levels more than low- to moderate-intensity running, which may explain why high-intensity running suppresses hunger more.

DO I REALLY NEED TO EAT STRAIGHT AFTER A RUN?

The longer you wait to eat, the less glycogen you store and the longer it takes to recover. There's a window of 30-60 minutes when the body is receptive to getting carbs back into the muscles. To know your carb needs, check your weight in kilograms. If you weigh 60kg, you need 60 grams (240 calories) of carbs within 30 to 60 minutes.

Your muscles are most receptive to reloading glycogen in the 15-30 minutes immediately following exercise because blood flow to muscles is enhanced during this time. Muscle cells can pick up more glucose and are more sensitive to the effects of insulin, a hormone that promotes the synthesis of glycogen by moving glucose out of the bloodstream and into cells. So it's vital to take in an adequate amount of carbohydrate – and protein – as soon after exercise as possible.

WHAT ARE THE BEST RECOVERY FOODS?

You may be able to boost the rate at which your muscles store glycogen, as well as speed up the recovery and repair of muscle tissue, by eating protein in combination with carbohydrate at this time. Drinks (liquid meals) are easier to consume when you're not hungry. Believe it or not, good old-fashioned skimmed milk is one of the best recovery foods out there. It not only provides carbohydrate and protein in the ideal 4:1 ratio, but it also has the advantage of additional calcium, riboflavin and magnesium. The protein in milk helps to rebuild muscle tissue and research suggests it may reduce exercise-induced muscle damage. A 2007 British study found regular milk is better than water or sports drinks at restoring fluid levels following a bout of exercise in the heat.

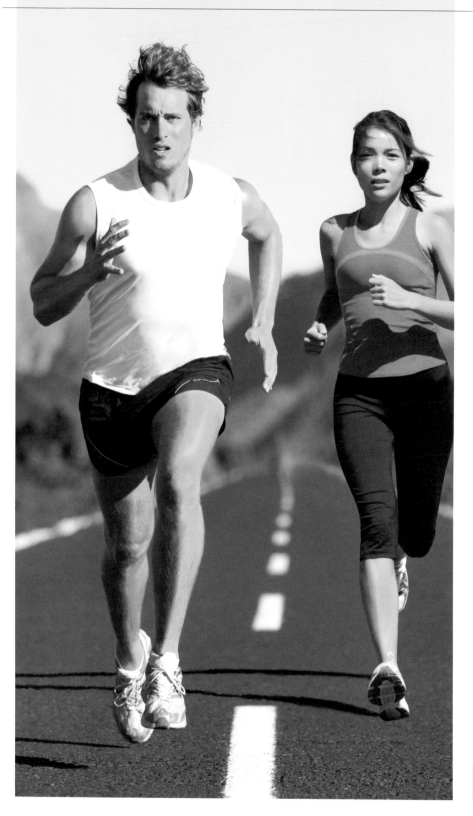

If plain milk doesn't tempt your palate, try a low-fat milkshake or low-fat flavoured milk. Flavoured milk has the ideal amount of carbohydrates and protein that tired muscles need for recovery. According to an Indiana University study, drinking chocolate milk post-exercise speeds up recovery and increases the time it takes to reach exhaustion during a subsequent exercise session better than sports drinks.

Meal-replacement products (protein and carbohydrate drinks) are also suitable, as are yogurt drinks and smoothies. Smooth and semi-liquid foods may be better tolerated than solid foods if you're feeling queasy after a run. Try yogurt, porridge, rice pudding, custard or puréed fruit. Bland foods, such as rice cakes or instant porridge, are also good.

'Although a low body weight is generally associated with better running performance, it's important to recognise that losing weight may lead to health problems'

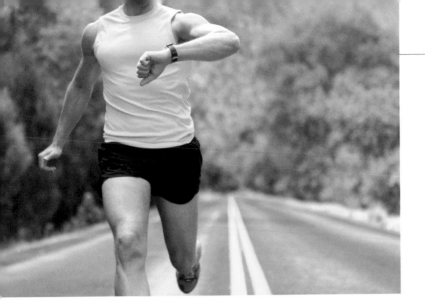

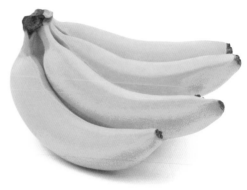

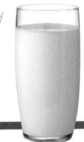

POST-RUN LUNCH

Not in the mood for a sandwich? These softer-textured options may appeal to your taste buds:

→ Lentil-and-vegetable soup with a soft wholemeal roll.

→ A couple of ripe bananas with two pots of fruit yogurt.

→ A large tub of rice pudding and a small punnet of strawberries.

→ Blackberry and yogurt shake: whiz together half a cup of oatmeal, half a cup of blackberries, two tablespoons of low-fat plain yogurt, two teaspoons of skimmed milk powder and four to six ice cubes.

POST-RUN DINNER

No appetite for a big meal? These healthy comfort foods may be for you:

→ Pasta mixed with cheese sauce.

→ Jacket potato with baked beans.

→ Cheese on toast.

→ Chocolate banana shake: Blend one cup of water, one banana, two tablespoons of low-fat vanilla yogurt, one tablespoon of chopped walnuts, one scoop of chocolate milkshake powder and six to eight ice cubes.

WHAT ARE THE RISKS OF BEING UNDERWEIGHT?

Although a low body weight and low body-fat level are generally associated with better running

performance, it's important to recognise that losing weight will not guarantee success and may lead to health problems.

In both men and women, being underweight can lead to an increase in illness, injury and fatigue, while in women low body fat also causes a drop in oestrogen levels. The threshold level varies from one person to another, but it's generally around 15 to 20 per cent. This fall in oestrogen leads to disturbances in the menstrual cycle and amenorrhoea (cessation of monthly periods), which can result in a loss of bone minerals and a reduction in bone density. In younger (premenopausal) women, this is called osteopenia (lower bone density than normal for age), which is similar to the osteoporosis that affects post-menopausal women, where bones become thinner, lighter and more fragile. Amenorrhoeic athletes, therefore, run a greater risk of stress fractures.

HOW TO GAIN WEIGHT SAFELY

Experts advise lowering the intensity and volume of your training by ten to 15 per cent and eating a little more. You may also need to adjust your training programme to include short periods of lower intensity training and more rest.

'Good old-fashioned skimmed milk is one of the best recovery foods out there'

TOP WEIGHT-GAIN TIPS

▸▸ Plan your meal and snack times in advance and never skip or rush them, no matter how busy you are.

▸▸ **Increase your meal frequency – eat at least three meals and three snacks daily.**

▸▸ Eat regularly and avoid gaps of longer than three hours between meals or snacks.

▸▸ **Plan nutritious, high-calorie, low-bulk snacks, such as yogurt, nuts, dried fruit and cereal bars.**

▸▸ Eat larger meals, but avoid overfilling.

▸▸ **Try nutritious drinks, such as milk-based shakes, smoothies and juices, to help raise your calorie, carbohydrate and protein intake.**

▸▸ Boost the calorie and nutritional content of your meals by adding extra dried fruit, bananas, honey, chopped nuts or seeds.

THE POWER OF PROTEIN

FROM AIDING TISSUE REPAIR TO BOOSTING YOUR IMMUNE SYSTEM, HERE ARE SIX REASONS WHY YOU SHOULD PACK MORE PROTEIN INTO YOUR DIET

PERFECT FOR PROTEIN

Four protein-rich foods for runners:

Sushi: Stay away from chocolate and crisps when you want a snack and opt for some sushi instead. Rich in protein, it will leave your energy levels stable and cut down your sugar intake.

Beans: Adding beans to casseroles, stir-fries, wraps and soups is a quick and easy way to increase your protein and fibre intake at the same time, helping to control your appetite, and aiding energy and health.

Lean white meat: Choose real turkey or chicken breast for a sandwich or wrap filling, instead of selecting sandwich meat. This has more protein and none of the stabilisers you'll find in the packaged variety.

Low-fat cottage cheese: This is a great source of casein protein, which will fill you up for hours for relatively few calories.

'Eating a protein snack after training can not only speed up tissue repair, but can also rebalance your immune system'

With the latest research suggesting protein can assist with appetite control, increase calorie burn and help you recover from your run more quickly, it's clear there are many benefits to be gained from having adequate protein in your diet.

1: FEEL FULLER FOR LONGER

Including a sensible amount of protein in your diet can help you manage your appetite. Not only has protein been shown to increase feelings of fullness after a meal, but when added to a carbohydrate-based meal it has also been shown to lead to more stable blood-sugar levels and a reduction in sugar cravings.

2: REPAIR AFTER RUNNING

Many studies show that adding ten to 15g of protein to a carbohydrate meal, drink or snack after training can reduce muscle soreness and assist with tissue repair. A lower risk of injury is also associated with regular protein intake after running. Simply add chickpeas to soup, choose a lean white meat for a sandwich or add nuts or whey protein to a post-run smoothie to benefit.

3: BOOST YOUR IMMUNE SYSTEM

As your calorie requirements increase relative to your running mileage, your protein requirements increase too. Not meeting this need can result in a weakened immune system, leaving you open to colds and coughs that could affect your training. Eating a protein snack after training can not only speed up tissue repair, but can also rebalance your immune system.

4: LOOK AFTER YOUR SKIN, HAIR AND NAILS

One of the many positive effects of getting enough protein in your diet is healthy-looking skin, hair and nails. If you're running on empty, the first signs can often be detected by looking at these visual cues.

5: INCREASE FAT LOSS

Diets with higher protein content (30 per cent rather than 15 per cent of calories) seem to have a protective effect on the muscles, leading to more fat loss and less muscle loss. Protein-rich meals also lead to increased calories being burned in the immediate period after eating. This is referred to as the "thermic effect" of food. In fact, a diet with 30 per cent of calories from protein has been shown to result in a three per cent increase in calories burned during the day, and even a lift in calorie burn during sleep!

6: IMPROVE YOUR METABOLIC AGE

Muscle generally declines as you age, which is paired with a slowing of the metabolic rate and a reduced need for calories. However, those who run regularly and include protein in each meal can reduce this muscle loss, maintaining the tone and muscle-protein levels of youth. With a higher maintained metabolic rate, you'll find it easier to lose weight and keep it off, and you'll benefit from a lower metabolic age.

STOCK UP YOUR FRIDGE!

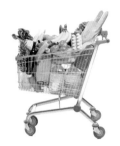

IT'S TIME TO DITCH FOODS WITH EMPTY CALORIES AND STOCK UP ON HEALTHY ESSENTIALS INSTEAD. THIS IS WHAT THE CONTENTS OF A RUNNER'S FRIDGE SHOULD LOOK LIKE...

1: STEAK (GOOD FOR IRON AND PROTEIN)

Steak is the ultimate meat for a runner. If you could only eat one type of meat, steak is the one you should choose. It provides plenty of protein, but also lots of easily absorbed iron.

2: SPINACH (GOOD FOR MICRONUTRIENTS)

This could be any green leafy vegetable, but spinach is particularly high in iron (though it also contains a compound that inhibits some of the uptake of iron). However, it contains other micronutrients, particularly micro minerals, which are needed for many processes in the body.

3: SALMON (GOOD FOR REDUCING INFLAMMATION)

Oily fish (including salmon) is a top choice for everyone, but especially runners. White fish doesn't have the same anti-inflammatory benefits because it doesn't contain the high levels of the omega 3 fatty acids EPA and DHA.

4: STRAWBERRIES (GOOD FOR ANTIOXIDANTS)

Strawberries not only taste good, but they are also high in antioxidants. Blended into a post-training smoothie, they will help to reduce muscle soreness.

5: BANANAS (GOOD FOR POST-RUN RECOVERY)

For a fruit, bananas are particularly high in carbohydrate and they contain other beneficial elements, including potassium and vitamin C. Add them to your smoothie for extra energy.

6: EGGS (GOOD FOR FAT-SOLUBLE VITAMINS)

Eggs are one of the most complete foods you can eat. They contain both essential fatty acids and essential amino acids, along with a myriad of vitamins and minerals.

7: PORRIDGE OATS (GOOD FOR DIGESTION AND ENERGY)

Porridge oats are an excellent, versatile source of relatively slow-digesting carbohydrate. They also contain soluble and insoluble fibre, important for gut health.

8: GREEK YOGURT (GOOD FOR DIGESTION AND IMMUNITY)

Research has shown that the live bacteria cultures used to make Greek yogurt can benefit both digestive health and immunity. It's also a good source of protein and calcium.

9: WHOLE MILK (GOOD FOR RECOVERY SHAKES)

Whole milk has been shown to be an excellent basis for a recovery drink, because it acts as both a rehydration fluid and also stimulates protein synthesis more effectively than lower fat versions with similar calorie content, meaning it's better for getting you back on track.

10: SWEET POTATO (GOOD FOR HEALTH AND ENERGY)

This is one of the best sources of starchy carbohydrate, to support your general health. Not only that, but its dark colour indicates its phytonutrient content.

11: BUTTER (GOOD FOR HEALTH AND ENERGY)

Butter is often frowned upon because of its high fat content. However, it's a good source of a range of fatty acids, as well as vitamins A, D, E and K. Remember to use sparingly!

12: HONEY (GOOD FOR POST-RUN RECOVERY)

Honey is a good source of high glycaemic index (GI) carbohydrates for filling up glycogen stores post-run. Add some to a recovery shake or smoothie for both taste and carbohydrate benefits.

13: TOMATOES (GOOD FOR ANTIOXIDANTS)

Tomatoes are well known for their high lycopene content. Studies have shown that lycopene can offer some protection against many cancers, including prostate cancer. Surprisingly, perhaps, the lycopene is more active in processed tomatoes.

14: PEPPERS (GOOD FOR IMMUNITY)

A red pepper contains more vitamin C than an orange. Plus, eating peppers with spinach will dramatically increase the absorption of the iron in the spinach.

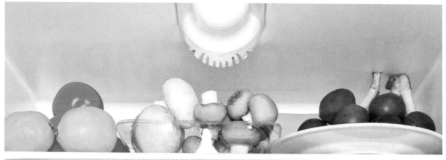
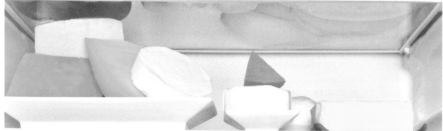
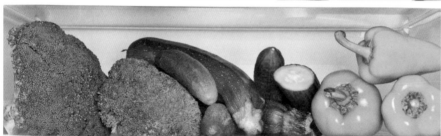
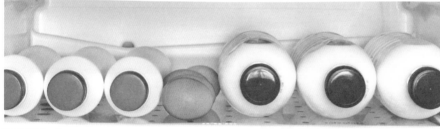
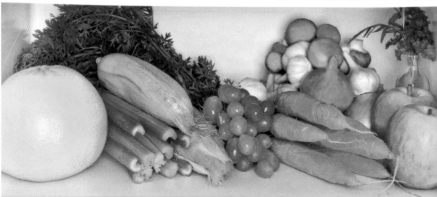

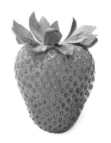

'Strawberries not only taste good, but they are also high in antioxidants. Blended into a post-training smoothie, they will help to reduce muscle soreness'

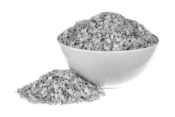

'Porridge oats are an excellent, versatile source of relatively slow-digesting carbohydrate. They also contain soluble and insoluble fibre, important for gut health'

RUNNING ON EMPTY

NEGLECTING YOUR MEALS IS NEVER A GOOD IDEA, BUT AS A RUNNER IT MAY BE GETTING IN THE WAY OF GOOD PERFORMANCES, AS WELL AS AFFECTING YOUR HEALTH

Is this you? You're a regular runner, but not really a regular eater. Maybe you can't face breakfast, then you're so busy during the day you forget to eat lunch altogether or you simply grab a quick snack. You tend to eat most of your food in the evening, so often you are running on an empty stomach. Perhaps you have chosen to run on fewer calories as part of your efforts to lose weight. If this *is* you, then you're not getting the most from your running and you may even be damaging your health.

FUEL FOR YOUR FIRE

When you run, your body burns a mix of glucose and fat for energy. The higher your heart rate, the more glucose (rather than fat) you burn. This is released from the carbohydrate stores (glycogen) in your muscles. The lower your heart rate, the more fuel you produce from your body fat. But even when you are running slowly, your heart rate is likely to be more than 60 per cent of your maximum, so glucose remains the major fuel source. Fat becomes the primary fuel source only when your heart rate is below 60 per cent of maximum.

If your glycogen stores are empty and you depend on fat for fuel, you'll probably find you can't run as far or as fast – it takes longer to convert fat into energy. You may also find it harder to recover from your run. This is why it's a good idea to eat some carbohydrate between 15 minutes and two hours before running, especially if you have eaten lightly earlier in the day and want to run in the evening.

HEALTH CARE

In 2009, the American College of Sports Nutrition published a paper in the journal *Medicine & Science In Sports & Exercise*, stating that adequate food and fluid should be consumed before, during and after exercise to help maintain blood sugar, maximise performance and improve recovery time. This is good advice. As well as affecting your ability to run well, regularly eating fewer calories – and therefore consuming fewer nutrients than your body needs – may affect your health.

If you combine a diet low in calories and nutrients with a demanding training programme, such as preparing for a marathon, you risk developing "overtraining syndrome", where your performance plateaus or declines, or you may become injured. In some cases, women runners who under-eat for a long time stop menstruating, have reduced bone-mineral density and develop disordered eating patterns.

THE FAST TRACK

As a rule, you should eat something before running, but some research has shown that people training for endurance events such as marathons may benefit from doing occasional runs in a fasted state, to increase their capacity to burn fat as fuel. This is known as "train low, compete high". But this approach has not been found to deliver performance benefits in shorter races, such as 10Ks, in which you run at a higher intensity and therefore rely on carbohydrates for fuel. It's not a good idea to do interval training or run for over an hour in a fasted state, and it's important to eat a recovery meal containing both carbs and protein shortly afterwards.

To get the most from your running, make sure you consume enough calories to support your activity levels. As a runner you may need more than the average (2,000 for women, 2,500 for

'It's a good idea to eat some carbohydrate between 15 minutes and two hours before running'

men), depending on your size and how much you train. Include sources of carbohydrate before and after your runs, and choose unprocessed foods, to increase the amount of nutrients in your diet. In short, watch what you eat, but in a good way.

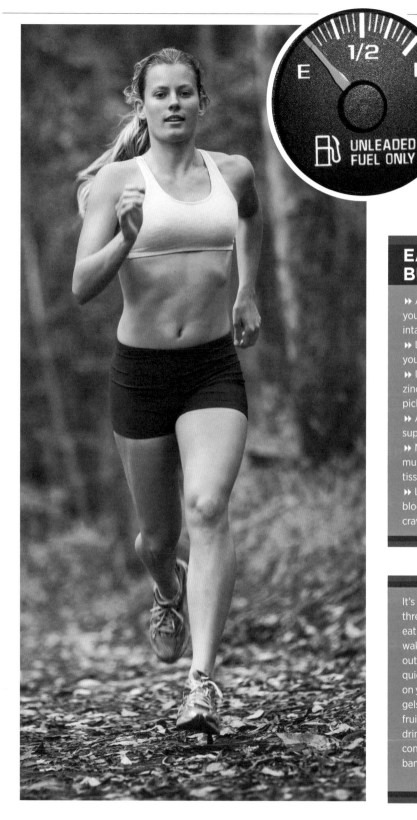

EAT WELL, STAY WELL. BUT EAT POORLY...

▸▸ A diet low in healthy fats and protein may make you more susceptible to injury, while a low calcium intake may weaken your bones.

▸▸ Lack of iron, magnesium or B vitamins may leave you feeling fatigued or lethargic.

▸▸ Inadequate amounts of vitamins A, C and D, plus zinc, could lower your immunity, raising your risk of picking up infections.

▸▸ A lack of carbohydrate during exercise suppresses your immune system.

▸▸ Not consuming enough calories could result in muscle loss, as your body breaks down muscle tissue to use as an alternative energy source.

▸▸ Leaving too long between meals could result in blood sugar imbalances, causing mood swings and cravings for sugary foods.

It's best to have a meal or snack no earlier than three hours before a run. If you have forgotten to eat something, or want to run shortly after you wake up, take an energy gel just before you head out. These semi-liquid sources of carbohydrate are quickly absorbed and you should notice an effect on your energy levels within 15 minutes. If you find gels hard to tolerate, a good alternative is a glass of fruit juice diluted with water, or 250ml of sports drink with a six to eight per cent carbohydrate content. Some people find they can manage a ripe banana shortly before running.

ENERGY &
PERFORMANCE
FOR RUNNERS

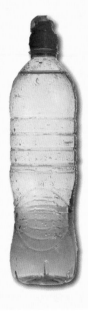

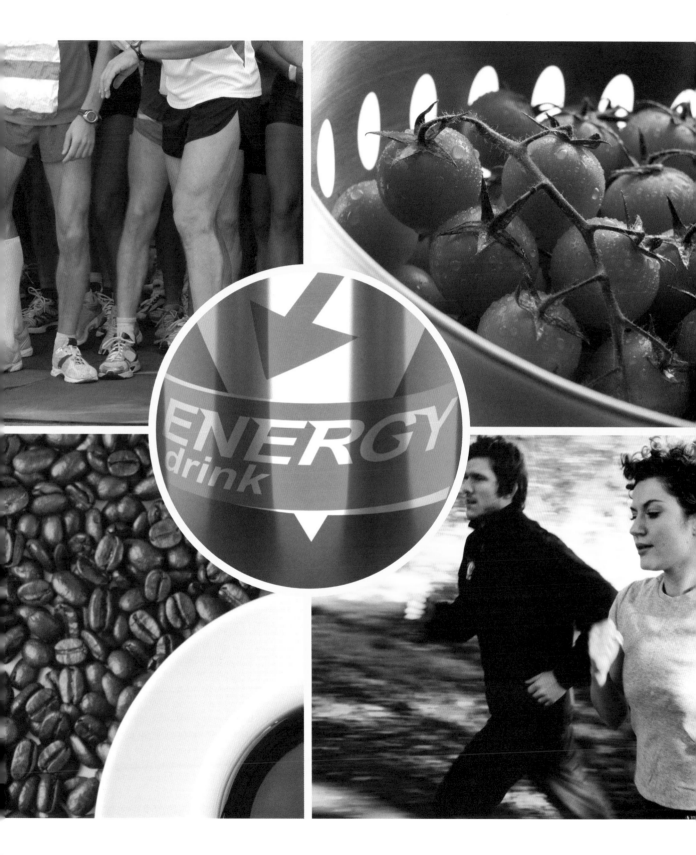

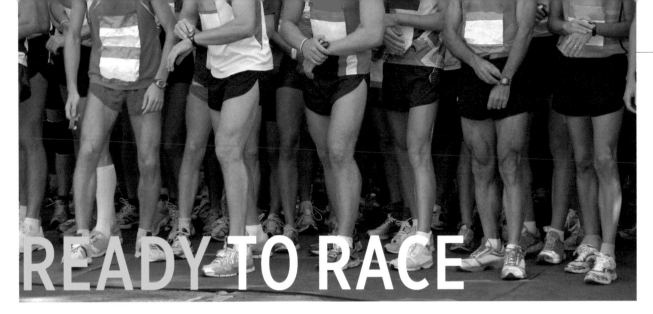

READY TO RACE

REGULAR CARBOHYDRATE-RICH FOODS AND DRINKS EN ROUTE CAN SUPPORT A FASTER TIME AND LEAD TO A MORE ENJOYABLE EVENT

If you're thinking of tackling a half marathon, 16-miler or even a full marathon, it's worth considering what you'll eat and drink on the way round. You've probably experienced running nightmares in the past – maybe you've eaten too much and continued to run with stitch-like symptoms, or perhaps you've hobbled through the latter part of an event, dizzy and tired, after consuming too little fuel.

Relying purely on water stops during long events will invariably lead to slower times, but equally it's no fun nursing a sore stomach as you drag yourself around. Wise race preparation will leave you feeling energised, focused and strong, but this means choosing the right food, and in the right quantities. Small amounts of carbohydrate can keep your batteries charged, helping you to run strongly to the finish line. Regular carbohydrate-rich foods and drinks can support a faster time and lead to a more enjoyable event.

FUEL CHOICES

Energy drinks
The most sensible choice for fuelling

your event, an energy drink provides both carbohydrate and fluid. Replacing between 30-60g of carbohydrate per hour in 500ml to one litre of fluid, this is the perfect way to stay focused and strong.

However, it can be hard to get a litre of fluid into your body in one hour in an event situation. Drinks belts, carrying bottles and hydration rucksacks can all be pretty hard to get on with. This is where more easily transportable carbohydrate sources can offer an advantage.

Sports Beans & PowerBar Ride Shots

Sports nutrition manufacturers have cottoned on to the fact that what you consume during an event is often dictated by what you can carry. Sweet-like carbohydrates, with added electrolytes to replace the salts lost in sweat, are great for drip-feeding the body with carbohydrate. Sports Beans (www.sportsbeans.co.uk) provide an easy-to-carry option, providing glucose as a sugar source, which is easily digested. They come in 28g packs, each providing 25g of carbohydrate, so are ideal to eat

slowly. Aim to consume at least 400ml water with each pack.

Eating a few at a time and sipping on water at each drinks stop should provide a good balance, but don't eat too many at once otherwise you could experience stomach distress. PowerBar has also launched a 'sweet-like' carbohydrate solution, mainly

HAVE A TRIAL RUN

Whatever your fuel choice, try it in training first, taking on board small amounts of carbohydrate once you've been running for 20 minutes. Ideally, sip on your energy drink or have two to three Sports Beans, a PowerRide shot or 1/4 to 1/3 of a standard gel every 15-20 minutes (you should be aiming for 7.5-15g carbs per 15 minutes with 200ml water).

Check out how far apart the water stops are spaced on your event if you're opting for a non-drink fuelling choice, as you'll need to wash it down with some water too. If you're choosing to wait a little longer to take fuel on board, be aware of the common signs of poor carbohydrate availability. Tiredness and dizziness are usually the first signs of low blood sugar, so watch out for these and take on carbohydrate immediately in small amounts, with water to accompany.

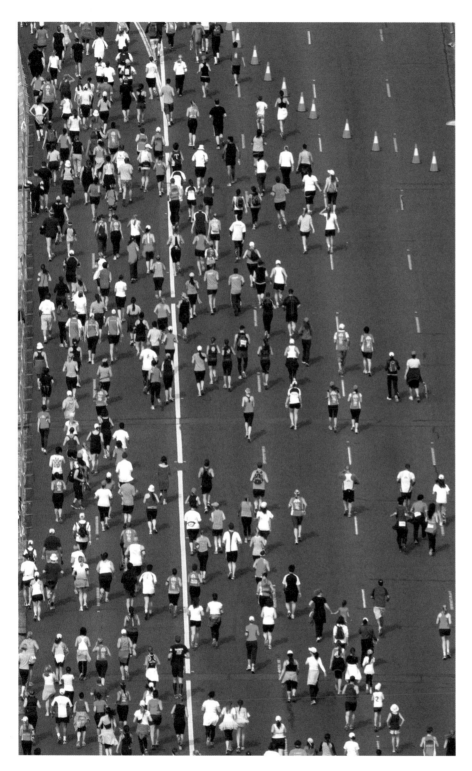

'Relying purely on water stops will lead to slower race times'

marketed to cyclists, but runners can benefit from the superior mix of carbohydrates, too.

PowerBar Power Gel Shots (www. powerbar.co.uk) are liquid-filled energy chews in a releasable bag. Ideal to clip onto a race belt, these super sweets provide a mix of glucose and fructose carbohydrate sources, found to encourage improved carbohydrate absorption. This mix of fuels has been suggested to improve performance by eight per cent, so it's certainly worth a go. They have no added colours, flavours or preservatives, but you'll still have to drink water to support hydration. For each half bag, drink 400-500ml of fluid. Less chewy than Sports Beans, these are an excellent choice for on-the-run nutrition.

Gels

Another convenient choice, sports gels provide a carbohydrate shot when you need it. Some runners have gastrointestinal issues with gels, but this is normally due to consuming too much gel with too little water. If you work on the basis that carbohydrates should ideally enter the body during exercise at a six to eight per cent concentration in fluid, then if you eat 30g of carbohydrate gel, you need to swig it down with 400-500ml water.

The trick with gels is to take them in small sips, with water. SIS Go Electrolyte Gels (www. scienceinsport.com) are hard to beat, coming in tasty varieties and digesting easily on the run.

EAT YOUR WAY
TO BETTER ENERGY!

WANT TO GIVE YOUR RUNNING THAT EXTRA BOOST? THEN FUEL UP WITH THESE TOP ENERGISING FOODS

WILD SALMON (FOR RECOVERY)

Salmon is an excellent source of omega 3 essential fatty acids, which are typically deficient in our diets. Acting as an anti-inflammatory, omega 3s may help soothe post-run aches and pains. Salmon also contains plenty of protein, important for muscle repair. Also, canned salmon contains plenty of calcium and vitamin D to support bone health. If you're choosing fresh

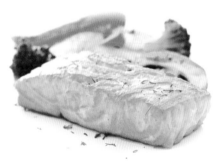

salmon, opt for wild Alaskan salmon, as it contains fewer toxins than Atlantic salmon.

Eat this: Aim for three portions of salmon each week for an omega 3 boost. A portion is about the size of your palm, or around 120g. Other oily fish, such as trout, mackerel,

sardines and herring, could also be used as an alternative.

BEEF (FOR ENERGY AND RECOVERY)

Not only a great protein source, beef is high in iron, important for women runners, who are often low in this energising mineral. Iron is required for delivering oxygen to the brain and muscles, so low levels can result in fatigue and may make you more prone to infections. Protein is essential for muscle growth, so if you want to increase your running power you need to ensure you're eating sufficient protein. An 85g steak contains around 20g protein. For maximum benefits, opt for grass-fed beef, which generally contains less saturated fat and more omega 3 fats, vitamin E and conjugated linoleic acid (CLA), which, studies report, may help reduce body fat.

Eat this: Include an 85g portion of lean red meat (beef or lamb) once a week.

CHICKEN (FOR ENERGY AND RECOVERY)

Healthy, low in fat and packed with protein, chicken is a perfect runner's food. A small chicken breast (115g) contains around 27g protein and all

the amino acids your muscles need for rebuilding, making it great for recovery. If you're feeling a little rundown, then it's worth knowing chicken is also packed with immune-supporting minerals selenium and zinc. And if you're looking for an energising meal, chicken provides plenty of B vitamins, including B6, important for energy production, plus iron to combat fatigue.

Eat this: For a great protein boost, aim to include chicken at least twice a week. One portion is a small, palm-sized chicken breast (100g).

LAMB (FOR ENERGY AND RECOVERY)

Lamb is an excellent protein-packed food, full of B vitamins, especially B12 and B6, plus iron for energy production and tryptophan to boost mood. The broad B-vitamin content of lamb can help support metabolism of carbohydrates – important to fuel your runs. Grass-fed lamb is also a good source of omega 3 anti-inflammatory essential fats, plus the antioxidant minerals zinc and selenium, which, together with its high protein content, makes it a great post-run food too.

Eat this: Include lean red meat (beef or lamb) once a week. A lean lamb chop (100g) contains around 20g protein and 208 calories.

TOMATOES (FOR ENERGY AND RECOVERY)

Runners can be prone to lactic acid build-up in their muscles following a strenuous workout. Eating alkaline fruits, such as tomatoes, can be effective in reducing this build-up. Tomatoes also contain a range of anti-inflammatory phytonutrients to support recovery. One of these, lycopene, has also been shown to support bone health in women. For optimal absorption of lycopene, eat cooked tomatoes drizzled with a little olive oil. As they're easy on the stomach and low in calories, tomatoes can help energise a run without bulking you up.

Eat this: Canned tomato juice is an excellent energiser, containing 4g of carbs per 100g, and the electrolytes potassium and sodium – useful before runs. One cup of cherry tomatoes (149g) contains just 27 calories, so include them three to four times a week.

PASTA (FOR ENERGY AND RECOVERY)

Pasta is an easily digestible food providing plenty of energy to fuel your runs. By combining it with a low-fat protein source, such as chicken, it's also an excellent choice for refuelling. Even if you're on a low-carbohydrate diet, including pasta before a long run can help increase stored energy (glycogen) in your muscles. When your glycogen stores become depleted, your body starts relying on anaerobic metabolism for energy, which may affect performance. For a slow-release option, choose wholegrain pasta and

allow two to three hours for digestion before your run.

Eat this: One serving is around half a cup of cooked pasta, which contains 110 calories and 20g carbs. Include this at least once a week before or after a run.

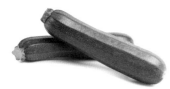

COURGETTES (FOR RECOVERY)

Courgettes are a great alkaline vegetable to combat lactic acid build-up, which can lead to post-run soreness. They are also packed with antioxidants to help support recovery and are particularly rich in the carotenoids lutein, beta-cryptoxanthin and zeaxanthin, known to reduce inflammation. The skin is particularly rich in antioxidants, so choose organic and leave the skin on. They're a source of carbohydrates including polysaccharides, which can help regulate blood sugar levels, making it useful for sustaining energy levels through the day.

Eat this: One cup of raw courgettes contains 4g carbs and 20 calories. Include them regularly through the week with a variety of other colourful vegetables.

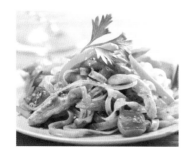

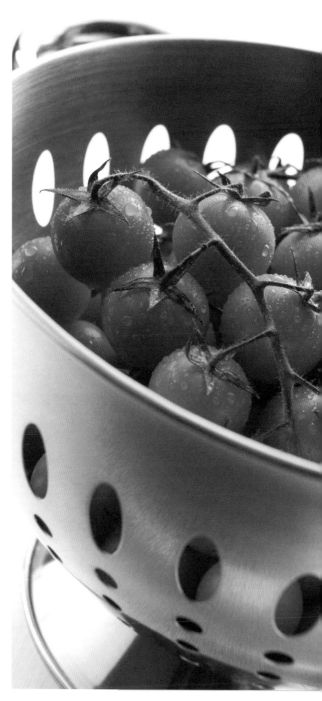

CAN YOU DRINK TOO MUCH WATER?

During long events, particularly those that take place in hot weather, simply drinking plain water can have serious consequences. This is because you're not replacing salts lost through sweat. This means that the sodium level of your blood decreases, which, in extreme circumstances, can lead to hyponatraemia. This can be serious, with typical symptoms including nausea, vomiting, headache and fatigue. As the condition worsens, confusion often develops and, in severe cases, coma and heart failure may follow. The simple message is that on runs lasting longer than 90 minutes, it's important to use an energy drink containing carbohydrate and electrolytes to keep the sodium concentration of the blood in balance.

THE LOO DILEMMA

Worried that drinking before you put your trainers on will leave you running for the loo? Include electrolytes in your pre-run drink and stick to 250–300ml fluid sipped slowly over the hour prior to your run. This will reduce urine output on your run and leave you sufficiently hydrated for the race.

'Dehydration will lead to slower, harder runs and poorer recovery'

GO WITH
THE FLOW

DRINKING ENOUGH FLUID NOT ONLY IMPROVES YOUR GENERAL HEALTH, BUT ALSO MAKES RUNNING EASIER

It's common to experience "dry mouth" while plodding the pavements if you haven't drunk enough water before your run. Feeling thirsty while running is uncomfortable and you can be left feeling daft that you simply haven't bothered to drink enough. But life can get in the way of those six to eight glasses of water you're meant to have each day, plus the extra you need to drink during and after running. Research in the *International Journal of Sports Nutrition & Exercise Metabolism* suggests even top athletes often start exercise in a dehydrated state. Get it right, though, and you'll feel better when you run, your performance may improve and your energy levels, skin and digestion will all reap the benefits.

WHY DO YOU NEED SO MUCH WATER?

Your body comprises 50 to 70 per cent water. You need to maintain this level of water with daily drinking and food to assist with growth, maintenance and temperature regulation. Not replacing enough water can leave you feeling lethargic and make everything feel harder, including running. If you run in a dehydrated state, your body kicks out more stress hormones. Your fitness can also be negatively affected – a study in the *Journal of Strength & Conditioning Research* indicated that lactate threshold, a measure of the steady pace above which you begin to fatigue more rapidly, is lower if you're dehydrated. Simply put, dehydration will lead to slower, harder runs and poorer recovery.

TWO EASY STEPS TO GOOD HYDRATION

Water balance is vital for health as well as performance, so it makes sense to have a two-step plan, one for your general fluid needs and one for running.

Step one: lifestyle drinking
The Food & Nutrition Board recommends you consume an average of just over two litres of fluid per day from drinks. This may seem a lot and might send you running for the loo at first! But your body settles down after the first few days of increased drinking and if you suffer from fluid retention, you should find that settles down too. If you work in an office, you may want to put a two-litre bottle of water on your desk and aim to work your way through it during the day. You should notice your energy levels improving if you've previously been under-drinking.

Step two: fluid on the run
If you're getting ready for a run and you've been drinking adequately throughout the day, you should have no problem working your way through a slow- to moderate-paced session of up to an hour without carrying any additional fluid with you. As you run, however, you'll be losing water through sweat. With sweat rates resulting in fluid loss of up to one-and-a-half litres per hour, you should try to satisfy this extra need by drinking up to 300ml before your run and 500ml on your return.

WHEN WATER IS NOT ENOUGH

For runs longer than 90 minutes, a carbohydrate drink can make a significant difference to your performance, so it's preferable to water. Indeed, research in the journal *Sports Medicine* indicates that sensible carbohydrate intake before and during your run can extend duration by approximately 20 per cent and improve performance over a set distance by two to three per cent. Selecting a drink that contains electrolytes is important for longer runs, as these are designed to replace the salts you lose in sweat. Taking on board electrolytes can benefit performance because they assist with hydration, but these salts also have a more practical benefit; they reduce urine output so you're less likely to need a loo stop en route.

GETTING IT DOWN

Physically drinking on the run will be your biggest challenge – you may find you get a stomach upset while running if you try to replace all lost fluids in one massive glug. Instead, aim for 250 to 300ml of a carbohydrate and electrolyte drink before setting off, about 800ml per hour while running and 500ml straight after you return. If you're out for a couple of hours, you may find it easier to run with a hydration backpack or bottle belt.

THE
BREAKFAST CLUB

LOOKING FOR THE BEST BREAKFAST TO FUEL YOUR RUNS? HERE ARE SIX TOP WAYS TO START THE DAY

Eating the right breakfast can make or break a run. If you run in the morning, you should ideally fuel up before you set off. This will give your muscles an energy supply to help you get the best out of your training, and it will fuel your brain to keep you focused and motivated. Plus, if you're looking to lose weight, it's worth noting that breakfast eaters – whether they run or not – are healthier and trimmer than people who skip it. This is because eating breakfast helps to balance your blood sugar levels, meaning you're less likely to become ravenous and overeat later in the day.

WHEN'S BEST?

Ideally you should eat something at least one hour before exercise. However, if you like to head out at sunrise, this may not be practical, so it's important to tailor your breakfast around your training. The suggestions here can be split, so you can eat a little before you head out and then finish your breakfast later. A mini meal of 100 to 300 calories is plenty for runs of up to an hour. So for the early morning runner, this could simply mean an energy gel with water, or a smoothie.

For longer runs – or if you run later in the day – aim to consume between 300 and 500 calories one to two hours before exercise. Whether you're calorie counting or not, the best breakfast combinations are those rich in complex carbohydrates, plus a small amount of simple carbs, high-quality protein and a little healthy fat. These breakfasts are tasty, simple and designed with runners in mind. So, if you need a little inspiration, these combinations will help you get the best out of your training…

1: HEALTHY AND WHOLESOME

Muesli is the perfect long-run fuel. The combination of wholegrains, nuts, seeds and dried fruit provides plenty of slow-burning energy, plus simple carbs to get your muscles working. Combine with milk and a spoonful of Greek yogurt for protein, and swap your milky cuppa for antioxidant-packed green tea, which has been shown to speed up fat burning and protect your muscles from damage.

TRY THIS: 60g Rude Health Super Fruity Organic Muesli served with 150ml semi-skimmed milk, a

spoonful of 2% Total Greek yogurt, a handful of berries and a cup of green tea. (Food guidelines: 317 calories, 42g carbohydrate, 15.8g protein, 8.4g fat.)

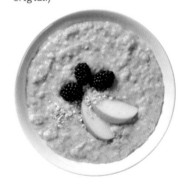

2: WARMING OATMEAL

Porridge is the perfect winter warmer for runners. Make with semi-skimmed milk for a creamy protein boost, or use half water, half milk for a lower calorie option. Stir in stewed fruit, banana or raisins for instant fuel. A sprinkling of cinnamon can help stabilise blood sugar levels, meaning you're less likely to suffer an energy dip later.

TRY THIS: 50g porridge oats or oatmeal made with 350ml semi-skimmed milk, ½ tsp ground cinnamon and 1 chopped banana. (Food guidelines: 457 calories, 70.7g carbohydrate, 19.4g protein, 10.7g fat.)

3: GRAB AND GO

If you can't face a proper breakfast or want to get out running quickly, don't miss out altogether. Try a quality energy bar with an antioxidant-rich smoothie for an instant satisfying option.

TRY THIS: Pulsin Energy Bomb! (www.pulsin.co.uk) – a high-energy product to boost performance. Add it into this berry smoothie: blend together 200ml pomegranate juice, 100g natural yogurt, 60g berries and 2tsp nut butter. (Food guidelines: Pulsin Energy Bomb!: 153 calories, 22.6g carbohydrate, 2.6g protein, 6g fat. Plus smoothie: 376 calories, 55.7g carbohydrate, 10.7g protein, 12.4g fat.)

4: SCRAMBLED EGGS ON TOAST

This is a great combination of protein and carbohydrate. Scramble a couple of eggs with a handful of spinach for an extra iron kick. Accompany with a glass of freshly squeezed orange juice, to increase iron absorption and give you an energising boost.

TRY THIS: 2 scrambled eggs with handful of spinach leaves, 1tsp butter, 2 slices wholegrain toast and 250ml freshly squeezed orange juice. (Food guidelines: 457 calories, 44.7g carbohydrates, 24.7g protein, 19.7g fat.)

5: A BETTER BAGEL

Choose a seeded or wholegrain bagel, for complex carbs, and add protein by spreading with low-fat cream cheese.

'Breakfast eaters – whether they run or not – are healthier and trimmer than people who skip it'

Top with thin slices of apple and a handful of raisins (dried fruit is nature's energy gel). Have a glass of coconut water, too – it's rich in electrolytes – to ensure you're properly hydrated.

TRY THIS: 1 wholegrain bagel spread with 1 tbsp low-fat cream cheese, topped with 1 thinly sliced apple and 1 tbsp raisins. Drink 250ml coconut water. (Food guidelines: 335 calories, 68.6g carbohydrate, 12.1g protein, 3.9g fat.)

6: FRUIT YOGURT CRUNCH

If you can't face much food first thing, try a simple combination of Greek yogurt, fruit and crunchy granola. Easily digested, it won't cause stomach cramps during your run. Pineapple is a great fruit option that's rich in bromelain – a natural digestive enzyme to help avoid tummy troubles. Greek yogurt is a good source of friendly bacteria and higher in protein than natural yogurt. Accompany with a glass of CherryActive – perfect for avoiding muscle soreness later on.

'Dried fruit is nature's energy gel'

TRY THIS: 150g 2% Total Greek yogurt, 80g fresh pineapple, 30g Lizi's Original Granola, 300ml CherryActive juice. (Food guidelines: 384 calories, 51.6g carbohydrate, 17.3g protein, 11.9g fat.)

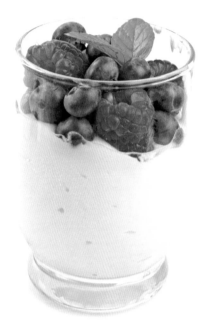

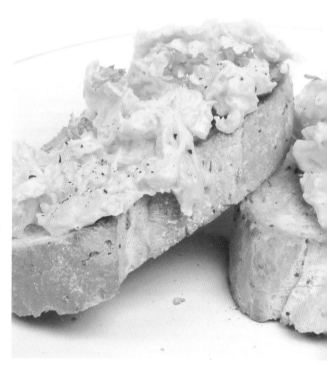

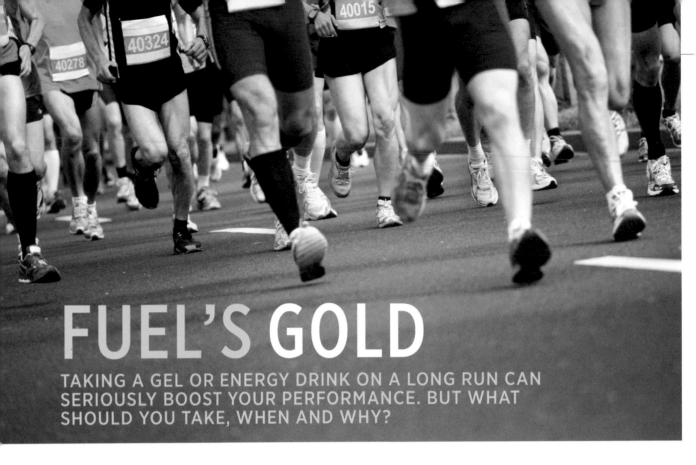

FUEL'S GOLD

TAKING A GEL OR ENERGY DRINK ON A LONG RUN CAN
SERIOUSLY BOOST YOUR PERFORMANCE. BUT WHAT
SHOULD YOU TAKE, WHEN AND WHY?

If you're new to running, you may have heard of energy gels, but have no idea what they are or how to use them. Or you may be wondering whether you should be using one of the many sports energy drinks on the market. If you're not sure how to use sports supplements to boost your running, read on to find out all you need to know.

ENERGY GELS

Semi-liquid gels provide you with a source of energy in a packet. Simply tear open and swallow while running. Taking gels helps to replace your carbohydrate stores, known as glycogen, which you use to create energy as you run. Gels help to maintain energy levels and enable you to run for longer, but should only be used when you will be running for an hour or more. This is because your muscles store enough glycogen to fuel your running up to this time.

The main ingredient in a gel is carbohydrate. This could be either the simple sugars glucose and fructose, or maltodextrin, a starch manufactured from glucose. Most gels contain a combination of carbohydrate types. This is because glucose and fructose are carried into your bloodstream by different biochemical mechanisms. Studies have shown you cannot absorb more than 60g of glucose per hour, but adding fructose increases total sugar absorption to around 90g, enabling more energy to be created.

Gels also contain some water, electrolyte minerals such as sodium and potassium, plus flavouring and preservatives. They may also contain caffeine, as this has been shown to benefit performance. Some gels are more diluted and easier to swallow than others. Most gels need to be washed down with water or they may not be absorbed into your bloodstream quickly enough.

However, some brands can be swallowed without water. Always check the label and make sure you stay well hydrated as you run. It's best to experiment with several different brands to see which you prefer, and do this well before race day, so you don't get any nasty digestive surprises.

'It's best to experiment with several different brands of energy gel to see which you prefer, and do this well before race day'

You can consume up to 30g of glucose or maltodextrin, or up to 45g of glucose-fructose mix per half hour of running. That's equivalent to two or three gels per hour, depending on the brand's formulation. Read the label or check out the brand's website to find out the recommended amount to use. It's best not to wait until you have been running for an hour before taking your first gel as, while quickly absorbed, the effect isn't instant. Try your first gel 30 to 40 minutes into your run and experiment to work out how often you need to take a gel during long runs.

Not everyone gets on with gels, with some people experiencing stomach cramps, tummy upsets or nausea when they try them. This may be because they have difficulty tolerating fructose, in which case it's worth trying a brand that contains only glucose or maltodextrin. Or they may have problems with the caffeine in some gels, or simply a sensitive stomach. Never try a new gel on race day!

ENERGY DRINKS

Energy drinks provide an alternative to gels if you're running for an hour or more. For shorter runs, stick to water or low-calorie electrolyte drinks, because staying hydrated is your priority. Like gels, energy drinks help to replace glycogen stores and their primary ingredient will be carbohydrate, together with electrolyte minerals. But energy drinks have the added bonus of giving you the water and carbohydrate you need in one product.

It's important to choose an energy drink that has been formulated for sport, with a concentration of 6-9g of carbohydrate per 100g of fluid. This will be shown on the label. Drinks such as fruit juice or highly caffeinated "energy" products such as Red Bull are too highly concentrated for use during exercise. They take longer to empty from your stomach and may cause discomfort, as well as failing to refuel you as quickly as sports drinks. Fruit juice may work for you if it's well diluted.

Sports drinks come ready mixed in a 500ml or 750ml bottle, or as a powder that you mix into water and carry in a drinking bottle. You can usually choose from tubs or sachets of powder.

It may be easier to use a sachet to start with, to ensure you're using the correct amount of powder. This will vary by brand, but it's generally recommended to mix one sachet into 400 to 500ml of water.

Aim to drink at least 500ml of energy drink per hour – more on a hot day. It's better to take several sips at regular intervals rather than take on large amounts of fluid at once, as this may cause tummy problems.

If you know a particular energy drink will be available at your race, practise using it in training, to make sure you can tolerate it. This will also give you confidence on race day.

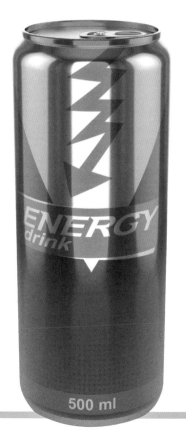

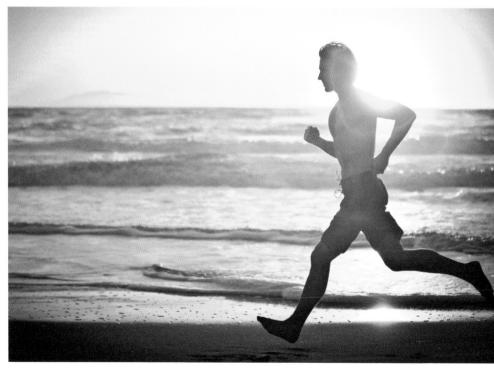

CAFFEINE AND RUNNING: THE TRUTH

IF YOU'RE LOOKING FOR AN EASY WAY TO INCREASE YOUR STAMINA, YOU COULD DO A LOT WORSE THAN DRINK A CUP OF COFFEE BEFORE A RUN

There is plenty of evidence suggesting caffeine improves performance in endurance sports. A 2004 UK review of 40 studies on caffeine and exercise concluded caffeine can improve endurance by an average of 12 per cent. And researchers at the Australian Institute of Sport found that athletes who sipped coffee or flat cola could exercise 30 per cent longer than those working without the stimulant. Another study, at the University of South Carolina, showed that drinking a cup of coffee before going to the gym delayed exercise-induced fatigue by up to 60 per cent.

However, before you order that shot of espresso, be aware that not all studies have shown positive results. Researchers at the University of Stirling, UK, and the University of Cape Town, South Africa, found that caffeine had no effect on performance during a 100K cycling time trial. And the benefits for sprint sessions are also less than certain.

HOW DOES CAFFEINE WORK?

Caffeine is known to increase your concentration, reduce the perception of exertion (so exercising feels easier) and boost your motivation to train. As a result, many runners find they are able to work much harder without realising it. It is also thought that caffeine triggers the muscles to use more fat as fuel instead of relying on carbohydrate. Because fat is in more plentiful supply, taking caffeine before a run can help postpone fatigue.

ARE THERE ANY SIDE EFFECTS?

For those who tend to grope for a coffee first thing in the morning, it's no surprise to read that caffeine is addictive. Even moderate drinkers get withdrawal symptoms, including headaches and fatigue, within 12 hours of eliminating coffee. Caffeine's side effects include anxiety, headaches, trembling and sleeplessness. Some people are more susceptible to these than others.

DOES CAFFEINE DEHYDRATE YOU?

Runners are often wary of drinking coffee before a long run, fearing it increases the risk of dehydration. But recent studies have challenged this long-held belief. In a study at Ohio State University, six cyclists consumed a sports drink with or without caffeine during a three-hour bike ride. Researchers found there was no difference in performance or urine volume during exercise, only when the cyclists were at rest.

In another American study, 18 healthy men consumed 1.75 litres of three different fluids at rest – the caffeine-containing drink did not change their hydration status. Numerous other studies have shown that although caffeine is a diuretic, if taken immediately before a run it won't dehydrate you or have a detrimental effect on your performance – in fact, quite the opposite. But at rest, caffeine drinks may "make you go" more frequently.

CAN CAFFEINE AID WEIGHT LOSS?

It's a myth that caffeine aids weight loss. Although it can elevate the metabolism (through its effect on adrenaline levels), this effect is very small and short-lived – not enough to result in significant weight loss. In fact, caffeine actually stimulates appetite and chronic consumption raises levels of stress hormones such as cortisol, which, unchecked, can lead to increased fat around the abdomen.

HOW MUCH CAFFEINE?

For most runners, the effects of a cup of strong coffee or a double shot of espresso before setting off should last throughout your run. Most studies have found performance-boosting effects with pre-exercise caffeine doses above 5mg/kg body weight – 350mg for a 70kg athlete, equivalent to three cups of coffee. But smaller quantities may work too, especially if you don't have much caffeine daily.

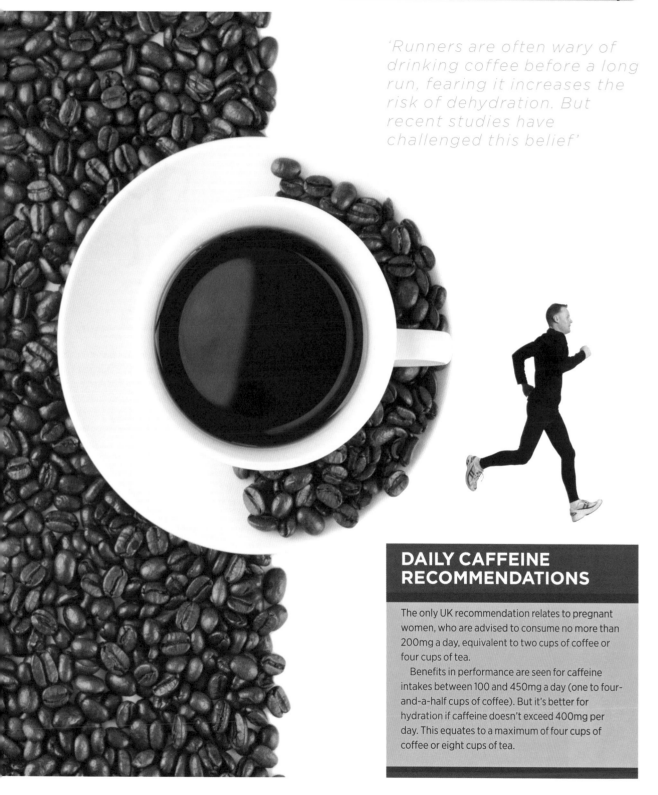

'Runners are often wary of drinking coffee before a long run, fearing it increases the risk of dehydration. But recent studies have challenged this belief'

DAILY CAFFEINE RECOMMENDATIONS

The only UK recommendation relates to pregnant women, who are advised to consume no more than 200mg a day, equivalent to two cups of coffee or four cups of tea.

Benefits in performance are seen for caffeine intakes between 100 and 450mg a day (one to four-and-a-half cups of coffee). But it's better for hydration if caffeine doesn't exceed 400mg per day. This equates to a maximum of four cups of coffee or eight cups of tea.

THE POWER OF ELECTROLYTES

THEY'RE ADDED TO SPORTS DRINKS TO AID PERFORMANCE AND BOOST RECOVERY BUT DO ELECTROLYTE DRINKS REALLY WORK?

The sports nutrition market is flooded with products claiming to assist running performance and recovery. In fact, there are so many that it can be hard to work out which products do what they're supposed to do and offer value for money. Electrolyte drinks, for example, are aggressively marketed at runners and endurance sport enthusiasts. But given the sometimes questionable claims made in the area of sports nutrition, you may well be wondering if you really need to reach for the bottle.

WHAT ARE ELECTROLYTES?
Electrolyte is a term for salts, specifically ions, which are positively and negatively charged. Your body's cells use electrolytes to send messages back and forth between themselves and other cells. They also regulate how and where fluids are distributed throughout the body. In short, we need them to live.

A healthy diet usually supplies an adequate amount of electrolytes. However, when we sweat, we lose electrolytes. These must be replaced to help restore body fluid balance.

HOW ARE ELECTROLYTES LOST DURING EXERCISE?
During exercise, your core body temperature increases because the working muscles generate heat every time they contract. As a result, you begin to sweat. This helps cool the body but that sweat contains electrolytes. The main electrolytes lost in sweat are sodium and potassium. Potassium enables the movement of fluids and nutrients across cell membranes, allowing them to carry on their metabolic activities, such as muscle contraction. Without sufficient potassium, muscles cells can't generate nerve impulses that control muscle contraction. Sodium also plays a role in muscle and nerve function and helps maintain fluid levels in the body.

HOW CAN AN ELECTROLYTE DRINK BENEFIT RUNNERS?
Electrolyte drinks allow runners to replace electrolytes, which aids the following:

→ Maintenance of hydration more effectively than plain water
→ Stimulates thirst and enhances fluid retention
→ Helps prevent voluntary dehydration

During post-exercise rehydration, the replacement of electrolyte losses is vital for the full restoration of fluid

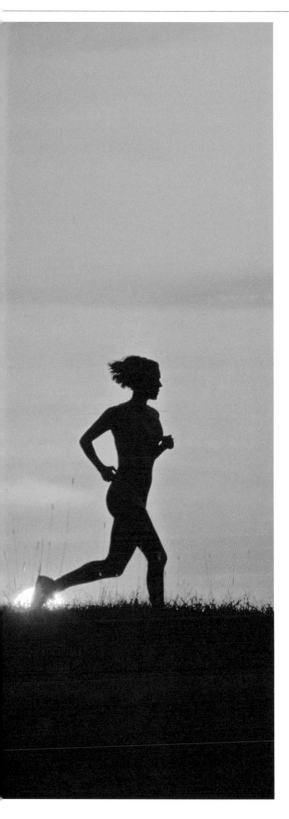

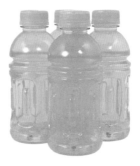

balance. Rehydrating with fluids low in electrolytes, such as water, can lower plasma sodium levels, causing a reduced thirst and increased urine output. Although you can replace your sodium by eating salty foods (eg, bread, breakfast cereal, pretzels), or adding salt to meals, electrolyte drinks with higher sodium content will more rapidly restore electrolytes. There is some evidence – although it remains in question – that whole body sodium losses may be a cause of specific types of muscle cramps in some people. Electrolyte supplementation may be beneficial in such cases.

WHEN CAN AN ELECTROLYTE DRINK BENEFIT RUNNERS?

Since electrolytes help your body retain fluids and may prevent muscle cramps, you need to replace them if you're running for longer than 90 minutes. You may also need to replace them with an electrolyte drink if you have a high sweat rate, are exercising in the heat or if you are taking part in a long-distance event such as an ultra-marathon.

ARE THERE ANY CONCERNS ABOUT USING AN ELECTROLYTE DRINK?

In some situations, excessive salt supplementation during exercise may lead to gastrointestinal problems or cause further fluid imbalance. It's vital that you practise using an electrolyte drink in training and not just in races, to get your body used to having it. Increasing the sodium content of a drink often makes it less pleasant to swallow, so make sure you take in enough replacement fluid.

SALT INTAKE

Finally, general guidelines for healthy eating suggest limiting the salt in your diet. Electrolyte replacement during and after sport may be a special situation but it's wise to be cautious if you have been advised by a medical expert to reduce the salt in your diet for health reasons.

'When we sweat, we lose electrolytes. These must be replaced'

RESTORE BALANCE

How much salt you lose while exercising depends on how hard you are exercising, how much you are sweating, how hot it is and how long you are working out. However, in general, if you're exercising for a long time or in high temperatures – when you'll sweat more – electrolyte drinks can aid fluid retention, stimulate the drive to drink and restore electrolyte balance.

GOING AGAINST THE GRAIN

WILL CUTTING OUT WHEAT AND DAIRY IMPROVE YOUR RUNNING?

Celebrities often extol the virtues of a gluten-free or dairy-free diet. Fine. Celebs often pay far more attention to their diet than makes sense, but when an athlete such as Wimbledon champ Andy Murray is avoiding certain foods – he has removed gluten from his diet – it's time to sit up and take notice.

But he's not a runner, you say. OK. But Paula Radcliffe is, and her gut problems were resolved when she removed from her diet foods to which she was diagnosed as intolerant. These included wheat (a source of gluten) and dairy. Furthermore, the Paleo Diet, known as the "caveman diet", which excludes all grains and dairy products, is becoming popular among those seeking to improve both health and sports performance. But does this mean you should remove gluten and dairy from your diet? Will it improve your running or could it have negative effects on your energy, stamina and ability to recover from training and races?

SHOULD YOU OR SHOULDN'T YOU?

Those with a medical diagnosis of coeliac disease, lactose intolerance or milk allergy have to exclude gluten or dairy from their diets. People who currently experience digestive health issues, such as loose bowels, abdominal discomfort, excessive flatulence or bloating, but have no medical diagnosis, may also see a benefit from excluding gluten and/or dairy. If your digestive health is currently good, you are less likely to see performance benefits from excluding these food types, although some people may. However, from a nutritional perspective, it can be beneficial to widen the variety of foods in your diet, so feel free to sometimes choose gluten- or dairy-free meals and snacks in place of your usual favourites.

It's perfectly possible to enjoy a healthy diet while excluding gluten and dairy products, so long as you make sure you choose largely natural, unprocessed foods, which provide a wide range of nutrients. The gluten-containing grains to be avoided – wheat, rye and barley – are good sources of B vitamins and magnesium, needed for energy production. This is one reason that pasta, made from wheat, is so popular with runners. Dairy foods such as milk, yogurt and cheese contain protein to help recovery from running and calcium to help maintain bone health. You will need to choose alternative sources of these nutrients if you exclude gluten and dairy from your diet. It's important to note that, while oats do not contain gluten naturally, they are often grown in fields where contamination with gluten is a risk, so you will need to choose products that contain gluten-free oats. Luckily, these are becoming increasingly available, as they provide a great source of nutrients for runners who need to exclude gluten.

CUT IT OUT

So, what should you eat to support your running if you are avoiding gluten and dairy? The night before a long run or a race, the following choices will provide a good mix of starchy carbohydrates, a little protein and a range of vitamins and minerals:

- Risotto, made with rice, chicken or prawns and vegetables (no cheese)
- Corn or rice pasta with chicken, vegetables and tomato sauce (no cheese)
- Baked sweet potato and grilled chicken
- Quinoa, steamed and mixed with vegetables and fish, chicken or a hard-boiled egg

▸▸ New potato salad with poached salmon

▸▸ Sushi selection (six to eight pieces)

Then choose one of these breakfasts, which should be eaten around two hours before you run:

▸▸ Gluten-free toast, with almond butter or mashed banana and honey

▸▸ Gluten-free porridge oats or quinoa flakes, with almond or soya milk

▸▸ Buckwheat pancakes with honey and berries

Or consume a gluten- and dairy-free energy bar, such as a Performax Sports Fuel Bar, Bounce Ball with Spirulina and Ginseng, or Pulsin' Energy Bomb.

After your long run or race, you need to replenish your carbohydrate stores and take on board some protein to promote muscle recovery, ideally within 20 minutes. Most commercially available recovery drinks and bars use whey protein, which comes from milk. The best option is to make your own recovery drink, using an alternative protein powder, such as soya isolate, pea or hemp. These are available from health food shops or www.pulsin.co.uk. Blend the protein powder with fruit and non-dairy milk, such as coconut, almond, rice or soya. Gluten- and dairy-free recovery bars include Maple and Peanut Protein from Pulsin', or Nakd Crunch bars and Trek Cocoa Coconut Protein Flapjack from www.naturalbalancefoods.co.uk. If you need to adopt a gluten- and dairy-free diet, follow these guidelines and you should be able to both run well and enjoy good health.

'It's perfectly possible to enjoy a healthy diet while excluding gluten and dairy products'

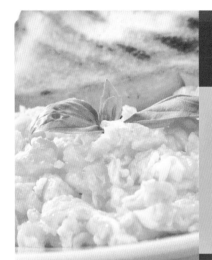

BEST GLUTEN- AND DAIRY-FREE RECOVERY FOODS

For optimal recovery following your run, have one of these meals within two hours:

• Kedgeree, made with rice, salmon, hard-boiled egg and rocket
• Quinoa or brown rice with chicken and avocado
• Scrambled eggs and mushrooms on some gluten-free toast
• Tortilla, made with potato, egg and vegetables
• Baked white or sweet potato with baked beans or tuna

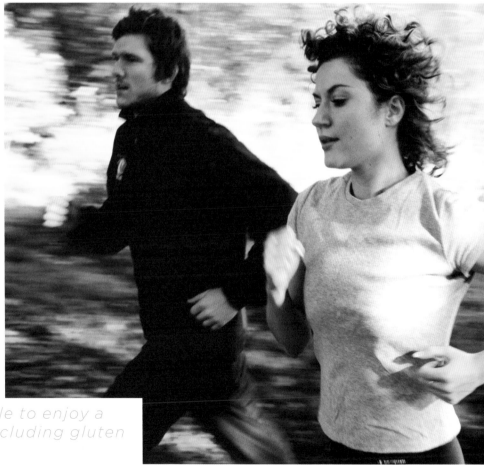

NUTRITION FOR RACES

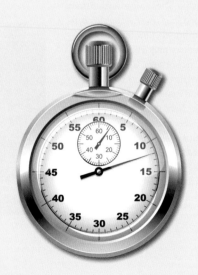

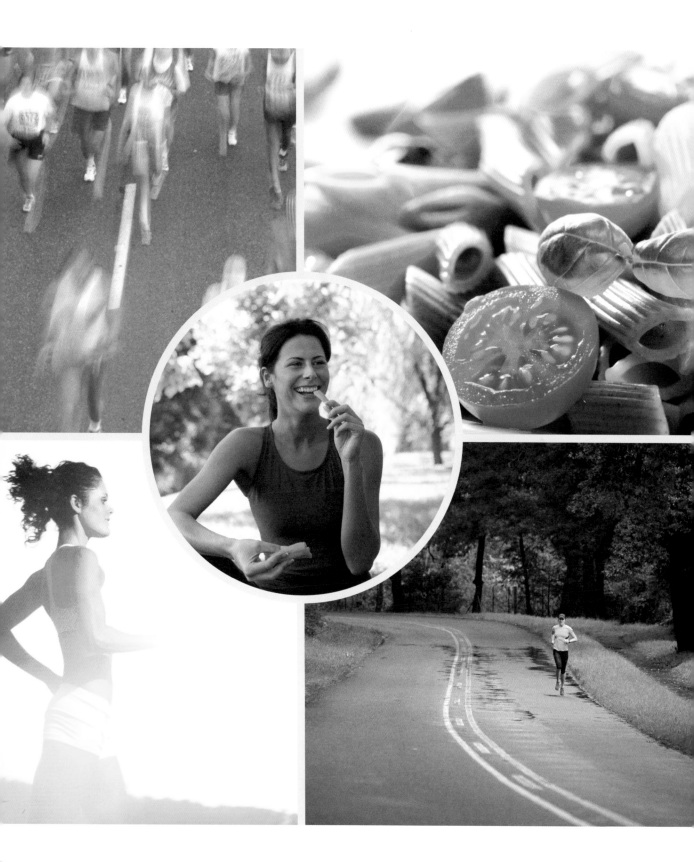

YOUR 5K NUTRITION PLAN

WHETHER IT'S YOUR FIRST 5K OR YOUR 50TH, GET IT RIGHT ON RACE DAY BY FOLLOWING THESE FAIL-SAFE NUTRITION RULES

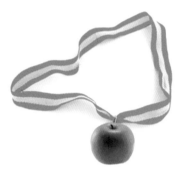

While you're training for a 5K race, eating a healthy diet should be an important part of your preparation. It will help to give you enough energy to run several times a week and to recover well between runs, so you are raring to go again. It provides you with nutrients to support your immune system, bones, muscles and joints, to help lessen the risk of illness or injury. And if losing weight is one of the reasons you are training for a 5K race, making the right food choices is as important as burning calories through running.

The amount of training required for a 5K race – typically three runs a week – isn't enough to justify eating more food than you usually do. There is also no need to consume sports nutrition products, such as carbohydrate drinks, energy gels, energy bars or recovery shakes, unless you are running for over an hour in particular training sessions.

Doing so can easily result in unintentional weight gain, as you may well consume more calories than you are burning on your run.

Instead, focus on the quality of the foods you eat and when you eat them. At least 80 per cent of your calories should come from high-quality, unprocessed foods, such as vegetables, fruit, wholegrains, lean meat, fish, eggs, pulses, dairy products, nuts and seeds. Only eat refined carbohydrates, such as white bread, white rice and white pasta, occasionally. Keep fried foods and fatty meats, such as chips, burgers, bacon and sausages, to a minimum. Watch your sugar intake carefully: not just treats such as cakes, biscuits, chocolate and ice cream, but also sugary items such as honey and syrups, sugar in tea or coffee, and hidden sugars in foods such as low-fat fruit yogurts or ready meals.

The timing of your meals and snacks is important on the days you

run. If you are an early morning runner, you may or may not run better after first eating a small amount of carbohydrate food, such as a banana or some yogurt, or having a few sips of diluted fruit juice. Take water with you on your run if it's a warm day. It's important to then eat a well-balanced breakfast within 45 minutes of finishing, containing both carbohydrate to replenish your energy stores and protein to help your muscles recover. Try wholegrain toast with nut butter or scrambled egg, muesli with Greek yogurt, or porridge with nuts and seeds. Don't forget to drink at least 250ml water to help you rehydrate.

If you are an evening runner, make sure you eat a carbohydrate-based snack around an hour before you head out. A banana, a dried fruit and nut bar, a slice of wholegrain toast with honey or a bagel with nut butter is ideal. Then eat supper within two hours of finishing your run – the

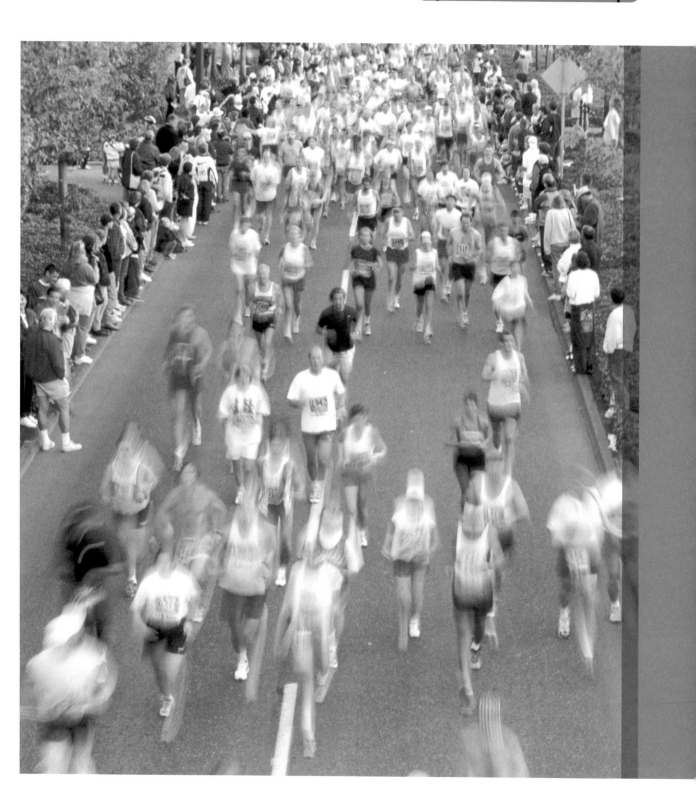

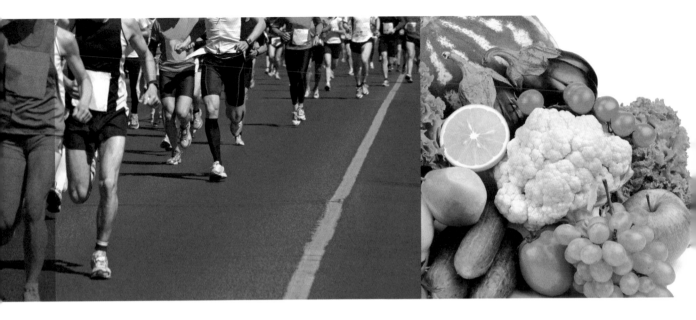

earlier, the better – choosing a wholegrain food such as brown rice, wholegrain pasta or quinoa, plus some protein from meat, fish, cheese or pulses and a large helping of vegetables. Finish with a piece of fruit.

Once you have your training nutrition sorted, you need to know how to prepare for the race itself...

THE WEEK BEFORE YOUR RACE

There's no need to load up with carbohydrates before a 5K race. In fact, doing so could mean you put on a few pounds, which won't help you run faster on the day. Simply follow the healthy eating habits you've developed in training and be careful not to overeat on your rest days before the race.

RACE-DAY NUTRITION

Be sure that you have tried out your race-day breakfast beforehand as part of your training plan, to be sure it isn't going to cause you any digestive problems. Eat around two hours

before the race, making your meal largely carbohydrate-based and with a little protein, but avoiding too much fat. It's also a good idea to avoid too much fibre, unless you are confident from trying this in practice. Try instant oat porridge with honey, white bread with honey or jam, a dried fruit and nut bar, or a fruit and yogurt smoothie. Drink at least 250ml of water. Have a coffee or tea before the race if you wish but only if you've practised this in training.

Be careful not to drink too much water in the hour before the race, or you might find yourself needing to stop for an unscheduled toilet break. It's best not to drink anything in the last 20 to 30 minutes before the start. During the race itself, have some water if you feel thirsty and if there is some available on the course, but there is no real need to drink.

RECOVERING FROM YOUR RACE

It's a good idea to have something to eat within 20 minutes of finishing your race. A banana, a bottle of

'The amount of training required for a 5K race – typically three runs a week – isn't enough to justify eating more food than you usually do'

chocolate milk, or a dried fruit and nut bar should do the trick. Keep this at the bag drop or give it to watching family or friends to look after for you. There is often something available in a goody bag at the end of a race; try to find out beforehand if this is the case and whether it will suit you. Drink around 500ml of water in the hour after your race; bottles will usually be made available by the race organisers. Then make sure that your first main meal after your race contains carbohydrate, protein and some vegetables to help promote a fast recovery. Salmon and rice, chicken and pasta, or a jacket potato with chilli or beans and cheese would all be suitable choices. Good luck!

MOTIVATION, INSPIRATION AND THE BEST WAYS TO IMPROVE YOUR RUNNING!

Every month, *Women's Running* magazine – the UK's only running magazine just for women – is packed with:

- Training plans
- Tips for beginners
- Recipes and nutrition
- Expert tips and advice
- Real-life stories

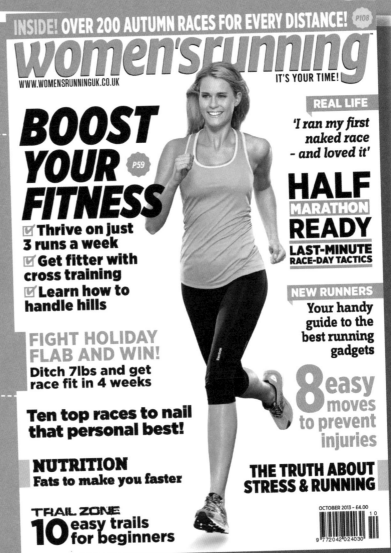

INSIDE! OVER 200 AUTUMN RACES FOR EVERY DISTANCE! P108

women'srunning
WWW.WOMENSRUNNINGUK.CO.UK

IT'S YOUR TIME!

BOOST YOUR FITNESS P59
☑ Thrive on just 3 runs a week
☑ Get fitter with cross training
☑ Learn how to handle hills

FIGHT HOLIDAY FLAB AND WIN!
Ditch 7lbs and get race fit in 4 weeks

Ten top races to nail that personal best!

NUTRITION
Fats to make you faster

TRAIL ZONE
10 easy trails for beginners

REAL LIFE
'I ran my first naked race - and loved it'

HALF MARATHON READY
LAST-MINUTE RACE-DAY TACTICS

NEW RUNNERS
Your handy guide to the best running gadgets

8 easy moves to prevent injuries

THE TRUTH ABOUT STRESS & RUNNING

OCTOBER 2013 - £4.00

9 772042 024030

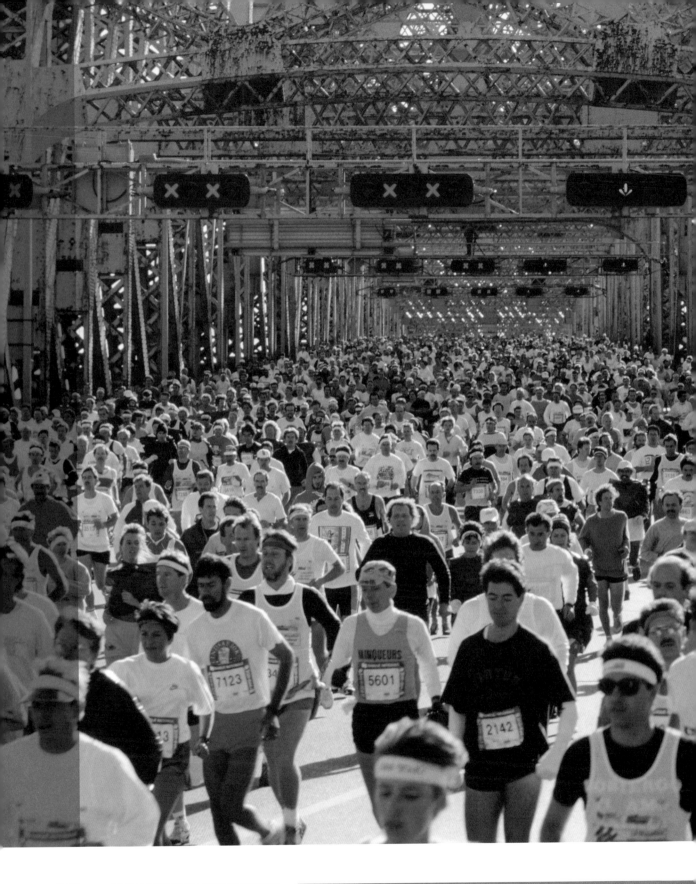

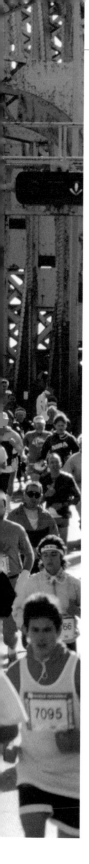

YOUR 10K NUTRITION PLAN

LOVED RUNNING THAT 5K AND DECIDED TO DOUBLE THE DISTANCE? NOW YOU'RE RUNNING FURTHER, YOU'RE GOING TO HAVE TO PAY CLOSER ATTENTION TO YOUR DIET

Whether you've entered a 10K race as the next step after completing a 5K, or you're planning to smash your 10K PB, you're going to need to start paying attention to what you are eating – and when – as part of your race-day preparation. Food gives you the energy you need to run and plays an important part in helping you to recover after you've finished your training sessions. The right food choices can also help to support your immune system, strengthen your bones and joints, and build lean muscle tissue. Your diet, in conjunction with your running, can also help you to reduce body fat, if that's one of your goals.

THINK QUALITY

Training for a 10K usually involves three or four runs a week. The harder or longer the run, the more attention you'll need to pay to your nutrition, maybe eating slightly more than you would on other days. This is particularly relevant for experienced runners putting in speed or hill sessions and running for over an hour once a week. But otherwise, focus on

eating quality foods rather than simply eating *more* food than usual. Your mileage won't justify the big increase in calories and you may find yourself piling on some unwanted pounds.

If you're an early morning runner, it's OK to head out on easier days on an empty stomach. This may help you to build your fat-burning capacity.

'On the morning of your 10K, eat the race breakfast you have practised in training'

Alternatively, have a small, easily digested snack, such as a banana, some yogurt, a fruit smoothie or diluted fruit juice 20 to 30 minutes before your run. You should always have something to eat first if you are doing a hard run or a session lasting more than an hour. After all your morning runs, eat a good breakfast – ideally within 45 minutes of finishing

– containing both carbohydrate, to replenish your energy stores, and protein, to support muscle recovery. Good choices include muesli with Greek yogurt, eggs on wholegrain toast, or porridge with nuts and seeds, plus a piece of fruit if you didn't have one earlier. If you do your longest runs at the weekends, on some weeks it's a good idea to eat breakfast about two hours before your run and to eat what you plan to have on the day of your 10K race. This will ensure your nutrition strategy is well practised, meaning you won't have any tummy troubles on race day.

REGULAR HOURS

Continue to eat every three to four hours during the rest of the day, which will help to keep your blood sugar level well balanced. Focus your meals and snacks on vegetables, quality protein foods, such as lean meat, fish, eggs, dairy products, beans, lentils, nuts and seeds, some wholegrain carbohydrate, such as bread, brown rice, oatcakes or wholewheat pasta, and one or two pieces of fresh fruit. Be sure to

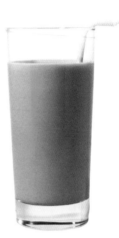

include some healthy fats every day, in the form of olive oil, avocado, nuts, seeds or oily fish (salmon, mackerel, tuna, herring etc). Keep processed foods, refined "white" carbohydrates, sugary foods and fatty meats to a minimum.

If you are an evening runner, eat a snack about an hour before you head out for your training session. Some dried fruit, an energy bar, a bagel with honey, or toast and nut butter is ideal. Then eat your evening meal as soon as you can afterwards – make sure this includes some wholegrain carbohydrates, protein and some vegetables. If it's been a hard session and you can't eat within 45 minutes, try drinking some chocolate milk as soon as you finish, then have your meal later.

When training for a 10K, you only need to use sports drinks and energy gels when you do long runs that last over an hour. Aim to take on 30g of carbohydrate during these sessions, usually around the 40-minute mark. That's 500ml of sports drink or one gel. Stick to water in all other sessions, or perhaps an electrolyte drink containing sodium and other minerals if you sweat heavily or if it's a particularly hot day.

So, now you know what to eat and drink during your training, what should you do in race week?

THE WEEK BEFORE YOUR RACE

There's no need to load up on carbohydrates the week before your 10K race. But do make sure your main meal the night before the big day contains a generous portion of starchy carbohydrate – such as pasta, rice or potato – along with vegetables and a small amount of protein.

RACE-DAY NUTRITION

On the morning of your 10K, eat the race breakfast you have practised in training, such as porridge, toast and jam, or a bagel and honey, and make sure you leave enough time to digest it – generally around two hours. Have a fruit and yogurt smoothie if you find it hard to eat breakfast on race day. Above all, try not to compete on an empty stomach.

Make sure you drink at least 250ml of water in the two hours or so before the race, stopping between 15 and 30 minutes before the start. You could also gulp some sports drink or try taking a gel just before the race starts, although if you decide on this strategy, do practise it before your long training runs. During the race itself, stick to water and drink according to your thirst.

RECOVERING FROM YOUR RACE

Make sure you get a good start on the road to recovery by eating or drinking something within 20 minutes of finishing – the sooner the better. Check out your race goody bag – it might contain a banana or an energy bar. If you aren't sure about what's

being provided, have something ready at the bag drop or with a friend or relative who's come along to support you. Sports recovery drinks and bars – which contain carbohydrate and protein in the 3:1 optimum ratio – are a good choice post-race. Alternatively, try chocolate milk or a sandwich with egg or chicken. Don't forget to drink enough water to rehydrate. The amount you need varies according to each individual; drink enough to produce pale-coloured urine. Finally, tuck into a well-deserved meal within two hours of the finish, making sure it includes some carbohydrate, protein and vegetables. Cheese and tomato pasta, chicken and mushroom risotto, or fish with new potatoes and green veg will all hit the spot. Go for it!

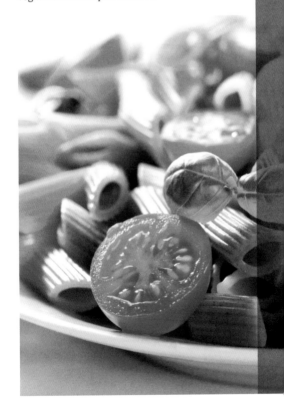

GET STRONGER, FITTER, AND FASTER AND NAIL THOSE PERSONAL BESTS!

Every month, *Men's Running* magazine – the UK's only running magazine just for men – is packed with:

- Training plans
- Tips for beginners
- Recipes and nutrition
- Expert tips and advice
- Gear and gadgets

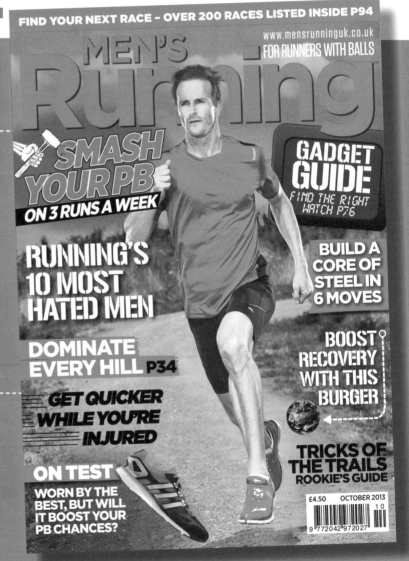

FIND YOUR NEXT RACE – OVER 200 RACES LISTED INSIDE P94

www.mensrunninguk.co.uk
FOR RUNNERS WITH BALLS

Men's Running

SMASH YOUR PB
ON 3 RUNS A WEEK

GADGET GUIDE
FIND THE RIGHT WATCH P76

RUNNING'S 10 MOST HATED MEN

BUILD A CORE OF STEEL IN 6 MOVES

DOMINATE EVERY HILL P34

GET QUICKER WHILE YOU'RE INJURED

BOOST RECOVERY WITH THIS BURGER

TRICKS OF THE TRAILS
ROOKIE'S GUIDE

ON TEST
WORN BY THE BEST, BUT WILL IT BOOST YOUR PB CHANCES?

£4.50   OCTOBER 2013

9 772042 972027

ON SALE MONTHLY IN ALL GOOD RETAILERS OR VISIT THE WEBSITE AT

WWW.MENSRUNNINGUK.CO.UK

FOR MORE INFO OR TO SUBSCRIBE!

YOUR HALF MARATHON NUTRITION PLAN

ONCE YOU'RE IN THE REALM OF SERIOUS DISTANCES, YOU NEED TO START TAKING YOUR DIET A LOT MORE SERIOUSLY, TOO

Focusing on what you're eating – and when – is an important part of successful half-marathon training. This is also the first distance where you need to take on some nutrition during the race. Read on to find out everything you need to know.

When preparing for a half marathon, you need to eat enough food to give you the energy to complete your training programme. This means increasing your meal sizes or number of snacks gradually as your mileage builds, particularly on the days you do long runs or high-intensity training sessions, such as speed work or hills. But, equally, there's no need to go overboard with your food. Eat too much and you risk gaining weight, which won't help your race performance.

Your food is your fuel. Choosing the right fuel will certainly improve your running and will also help your muscles to recover more quickly after training, reduce the level of fatigue you experience and also reduce your risk of succumbing to a cold or other infection.

Carbohydrates provide the major source of energy for training and should make up 45-55 per cent of the calories in your diet. Before you run, eat some quickly absorbed carbohydrate from fruit, fruit juice, dried fruit, energy bars or yogurt.

Your meals should include complex carbohydrates that provide slower-

'Your food is your fuel. Choosing the right fuel will certainly improve your running'

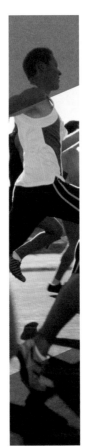

released but longer-lasting energy. A good amount should come from vegetables, including sweet potatoes and pulses such as beans, lentils and chickpeas, with the remainder coming from wholegrain or rye bread, wholewheat pasta, brown or basmati rice, porridge oats, oatcakes, quinoa or wholewheat

couscous. Try to eat two to four portions of fruit each day too.

Aim to have some protein in every meal and in most snacks. Protein helps your muscles to recover from training and supports your immune system. It's particularly important to include some protein in your post-run recovery snack or meal, alongside carbohydrate. This can come from the protein that's usually an ingredient in recovery drinks and bars, but can also come from food sources such as meat, fish, eggs, dairy products, nuts, seeds, beans and lentils.

Try making your own smoothies with fruit and yogurt, have a turkey salad sandwich or try some sushi. Many people don't include protein at breakfast; this is particularly important for effective recovery if you've done an early morning run, and will help to keep your blood sugar – and therefore your energy levels – better balanced throughout the day. Try adding nuts to your porridge, yogurt to muesli, and eating eggs or almond butter on toast.

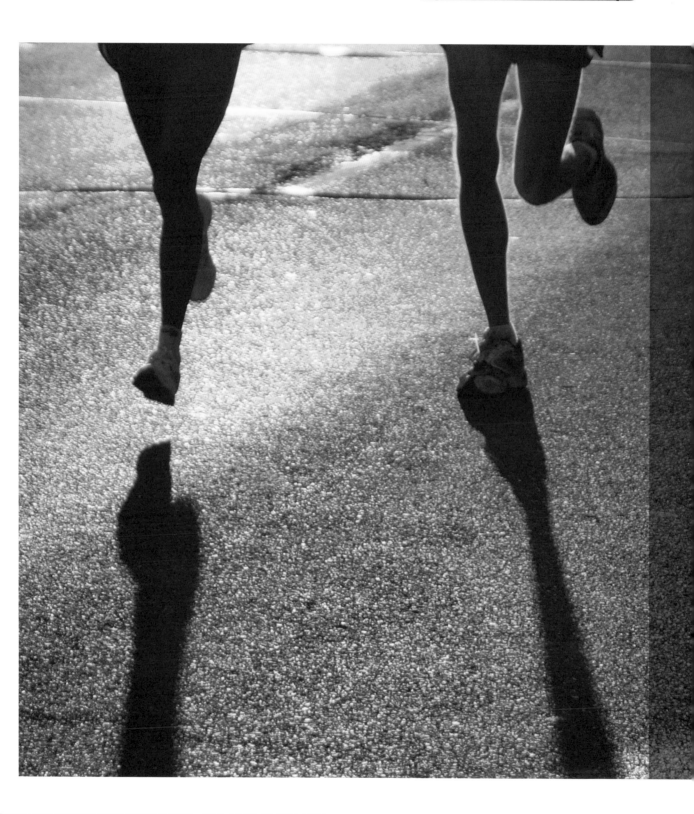

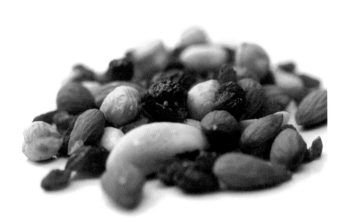

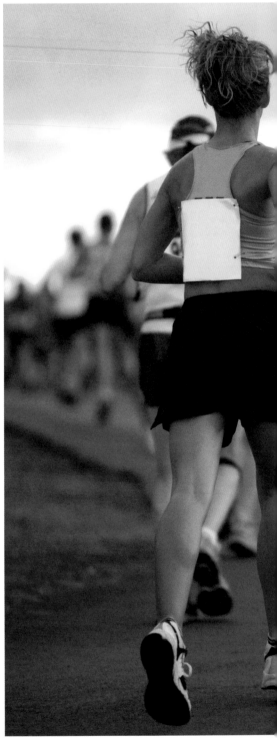

Don't forget to include some healthy fats in your diet. They are important for your immune system and heart health, while also providing part of the fuel you burn on lower intensity runs. Oily fish, such as salmon and mackerel, a variety of nuts and seeds, avocado, dairy products, olive oil and coconut oil will provide you with a good range of fats. However, it's best to avoid foods high in fat just before running if you have a sensitive stomach.

Once your long runs are lasting for more than an hour, you'll need to replenish your carbohydrate stores, known as muscle glycogen, while you run. The best way to do this is to use energy gels or a specially formulated sports drink, which should also contain electrolytes, including sodium and potassium. Some gels also contain caffeine. One gel or 500ml of sports drink will give you 30g of quickly absorbed carbohydrate from glucose, fructose or maltodextrin. Most runners need between 30g and 60g per hour to keep their glycogen topped up. It's important to practise this strategy before your race. Find out which

brand will be available on race day and see if it works well for you. If not, you'll need to carry your own choice. Here's how to prepare in the final seven days before your half marathon, and on the day itself…

THE WEEK BEFORE YOUR RACE

There's no need to eat a lot of extra carbohydrate in the days before you race a half marathon – it could cause weight gain. But over the last week, as you reduce your training mileage, look to eat a little less protein and fat than usual and a little more carbohydrate. An extra spoonful of rice, an additional slice of bread or another potato is all you need. Do make sure you have a carbohydrate-rich meal the night before your race, without having too much fibre or fat in case it upsets your stomach. Pasta or risotto make great pre-race dinner choices.

RACE-DAY NUTRITION

Eat your pre-race breakfast about two hours before the race starts. This needs to provide energy quickly, so opt for white bread, instant porridge or an energy bar. Have a smoothie if you can't face solid food. Make sure you have practised your race-day breakfast in training. Drink at least 250ml of water before the race, stopping between 15 and 30 minutes before the start to allow a final toilet visit. Then take a gel and a little water, or about 100ml of sports drink, in the final five minutes before the start.

During the race, you will need to use your own energy gels or the sports drink provided. The amount you need will depend on the pace you are running at and how well you can absorb the carbohydrate. Work out a practicable refuelling plan beforehand. A 30g energy gel every 30 minutes is a typical strategy, washed down with water provided on the course. Alternatively, know at what points a sports drink will be provided and take advantage of that. Drink additional water according to your thirst.

RECOVERING FROM YOUR RACE

Eat or drink something within 20 minutes of the race finishing – the sooner the better. There may be a piece of fruit or an energy bar provided at the finish, or make sure

you have something available at the bag drop or with a supporter.

Recovery drinks containing carbohydrate and protein work well after races, as they both rehydrate and give you the nutrition you need. Then eat a meal within two hours of the finish, making sure this includes some carbohydrate – such as bread, rice, pasta or potatoes – some vegetables, and some protein from meat, fish or cheese. You may then need another snack two hours later, particularly if you feel fatigued or lightheaded. Don't forget to drink at least a litre of water during the hours after the race too.

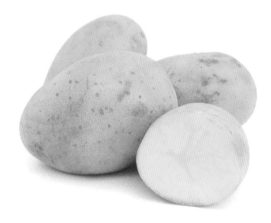

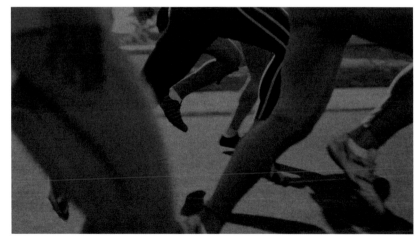

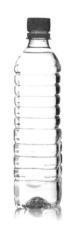

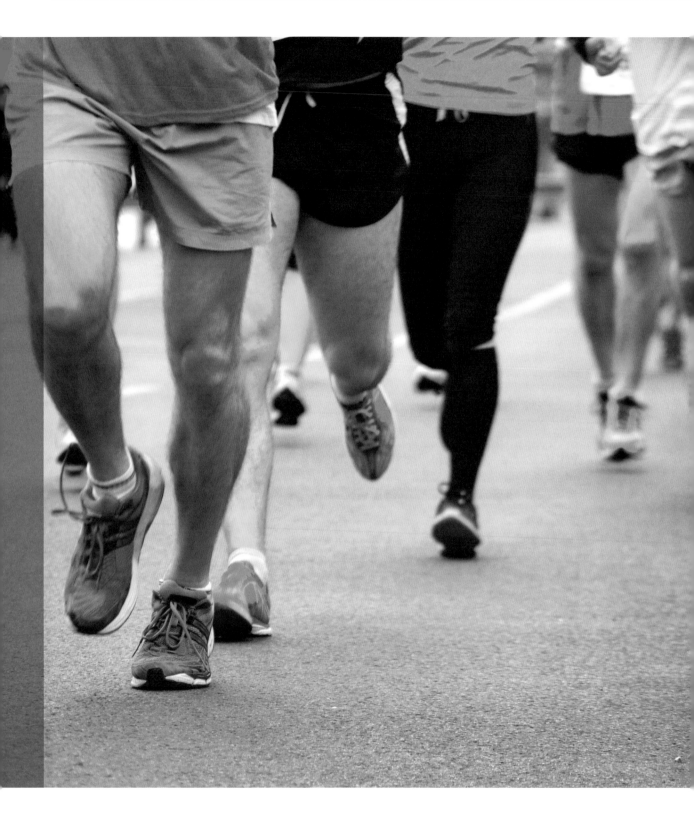

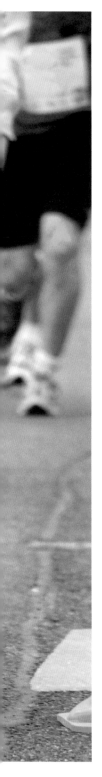

YOUR MARATHON NUTRITION PLAN

MAKE SURE YOUR DIET WILL HELP YOU GO THE DISTANCE WHEN YOU TAKE ON THAT 26.2-MILE CHALLENGE

The amount and quality of the food you eat – and when you eat it – have a significant role to play in training for and completing a marathon. As your weekly training mileage builds, you should plan how your diet will change to support all the effort you are making. Not taking

'Training for a marathon with weight loss as your main goal is most certainly not a good idea'

on board enough calories and nutrients to fuel your heavy training and facilitate your recovery is a classic mistake, and one that could contribute to overtraining syndrome, where your progress stalls as a result of fatigue, lack of motivation and possibly injury or illness. Training

for a marathon with weight loss as your main goal is most certainly not a good idea.

The first area to consider is your carbohydrate intake. Carbs are your main source of fuel for running, although you also obtain some energy from fat stores. Carbs are

broken down to glucose and stored in your muscles in the form of glycogen. These stores are limited, and you need to top them up both before and after running. The more miles you run, the higher your carbohydrate needs are. So, you should be eating more carbohydrate as you progress in

your training plan. Also, bear in mind that the heavier you are, the more carbs you will need. Consuming 4-6g per kilogram of body weight in your everyday diet is a useful guide. You can use a food diary app, such as MyFitnessPal, to track this. In addition, you'll need to obtain quickly absorbed carbs, such as glucose, fructose or maltodextrin, from energy gels and sports drinks during your long runs. These should also contain electrolytes, including sodium or potassium, to replace those lost in sweat. Aim to consume between 30g and 60g of carbs per hour of running on these long-distance days, and practise with the products you will use while running the marathon itself. Within 20 minutes of finishing your run, eat or drink some carbohydrate and protein to help kick-start your recovery. Chocolate milk works well.

Follow this with a good meal within two hours of finishing.

The majority of your carbs should come from natural sources: think vegetables, fruit and wholegrains, such as wholemeal bread, rye bread, oats, wholewheat pasta and brown rice. This will also give you plenty of fibre and provide you with slow-release energy.

Before you run, however, it's best to choose carbs that release energy more quickly and contain less fibre. White bread or bagels, white rice or pasta, rice cakes or an energy bar are all good examples of pre-run snacks if you are heading out for an evening run. If you run before breakfast, have a banana or drink some diluted fruit juice first if you are doing a hard session such as hills, intervals or tempo. If it's a slower paced short run, you may prefer to not eat or drink anything. It is very important, however, to eat a good-quality breakfast every day, whether you have a run or not. This should include some wholegrains and some protein, such as eggs, yogurt or nut butter.

As well as carbohydrates, you need to think about your protein and fat

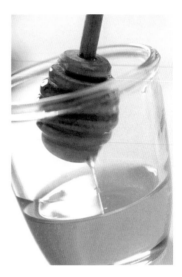

intake. Protein helps your muscles to recover from training and supports your immune system. Lean meat, fish, eggs, dairy products, pulses, nuts and seeds all provide protein, and it's a good idea to include some in every meal and snack. It's also important when you're training for a marathon to include some good-quality fats in your diet, such as avocado, olive oil, nuts and oily fish, such as salmon or mackerel. These fats play a number of important roles in maintaining your health, including supporting your immune system. Lastly, while the odd treat is fine, keep foods such as cakes, biscuits, pastries, ice cream and fatty, processed meats to a minimum, or you may gain weight despite all your training.

THE WEEK BEFORE YOUR RACE

As you start your taper, you should reduce the amount of carbohydrate in your diet in line with your reduced mileage, or you risk weight gain before your race. However, three days before your marathon, start the carbohydrate-loading process to ensure your glycogen stores are full

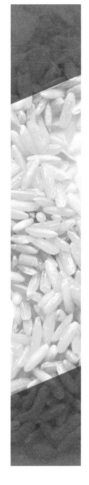

on your big day. This doesn't mean eating more calories overall, but making starchy and sugary foods a bigger proportion of your diet than normal, and cutting back on protein and fat. As well as eating bread, pasta, rice and potatoes, use fruit juices, fruit smoothies, jams, honey and energy bars to get your extra carbs. Make sure you have tried out your pre-race dinner the night before one of your long runs, and keep it low in fat, fibre and spices, to prevent unwanted tummy problems during the race. It's a good idea to eat no later than 7pm.

RACE-DAY NUTRITION

It's essential to practise your pre-race breakfast strategy on a long run in training. Have a tried-and-tested breakfast at least two hours before the marathon start time. For some people, who can handle some fibre, this might be porridge and banana; for others, it will be white toast and jam or a bagel with honey. For some, a simple fruit smoothie or sports drink may be all they can manage. Drink around 500ml of water in the hour or two before the start, stopping in time to have a last toilet visit.

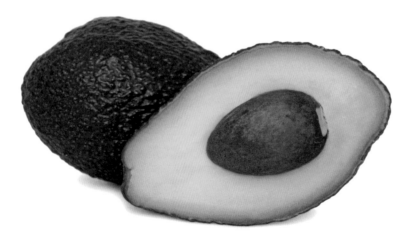

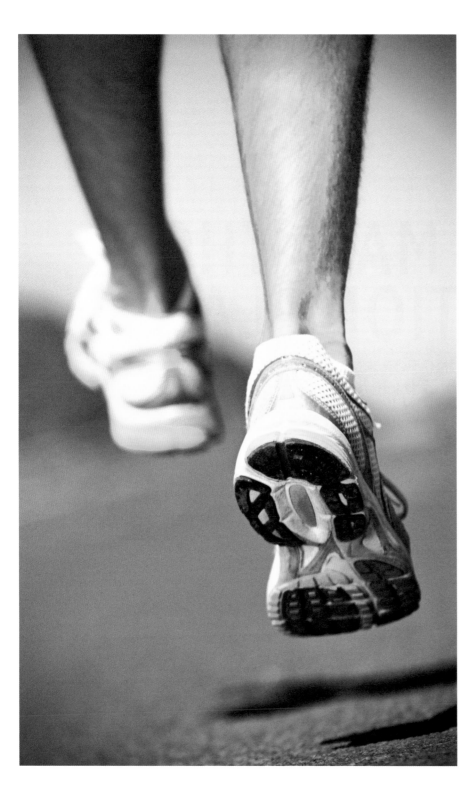

Finally, take an energy gel and a little water or a few sips of sports drink ten to 15 minutes before you start the race.

During the race, use the fuelling and hydration strategy that you have practised on your long runs. This might mean using the sports drink provided – check beforehand where on the course this will be found – or carrying your own gels and using the water provided to wash them down. Again, know where the water points will be. Don't leave it more than an hour before first taking on some energy replenishment. Ideally, plan how much you will take on board and when you will do it. You also need to keep yourself well hydrated with water, but use your thirst as a guide. Drinking too much dilutes the sodium levels in your blood and can result in a dangerous medical condition called hyponatraemia. Symptoms include nausea and vomiting, confusion, headaches and, in severe cases, loss of consciousness and coma.

RECOVERING FROM YOUR RACE

Getting your nutrition right after your marathon is almost as important as having the correct refuelling strategy during the race. Plan ahead, to make sure you have access to your favourite recovery product, and use it within 20 minutes of finishing. Keep it at the bag drop or with a supporter. Drink 500ml to 1,000ml of water in the first hour after the race and keep drinking until your urine is pale. Enjoy your post-run meal within two hours, but make sure it contains some carbs, protein and vegetables. Then have a further snack or recovery drink about two hours later, to prevent an energy crash. If you're struggling to eat solid foods, flavoured milk or fruit yogurt are good options.

YOUR ULTRA MARATHON NUTRITION PLAN

WHEN YOU'RE TRAINING FOR AN ULTRA MARATHON, IT'S NOT UNCOMMON TO BE OUT RUNNING FOR HOURS AT A TIME, SO GOOD NUTRITION IS ABSOLUTELY KEY

If you've decided to run an ultra marathon, you've almost certainly run at least one marathon-distance race before. And if well-planned nutrition is important for succeeding in a marathon, it's even more vital when moving up to ultra distances, whether it's 28 or 65 miles, or more. Not only will your training load increase to enable you to cope with a longer race distance, but you will also need a different nutritional strategy for the race itself, which is likely to include solid food as well as gels and sports drinks.

There are two main differences in the training plans undertaken by ultra runners and those training for a marathon. The first is that you will probably run twice on some days of the week. The second is that you are likely to be doing more than one long run (90 minutes or more) each week. Both add up to more running volume and therefore require extra nutritional support. The basic principles of a healthy diet for runners still apply, of course. You need to eat enough food to support your training, you need a wide range of foods in your diet to provide plenty of different nutrients to support good health, and you should aim to eat unprocessed foods most of the time.

Around half your calories will be from carbohydrates, most of which should come from complex carbs, such as wholegrains, vegetables and pulses, which release energy slowly. Some will come from natural sugars found in fruit, from quick-releasing starches in refined carbs, such as white bread (before runs) or from added sugars in sports drinks, energy bars, gels and recovery products, particularly on your harder training days. Try to include five to six portions of vegetables and three to four portions of fruit in your diet every day.

You should also include some protein in every meal and most snacks, particularly after training sessions. Protein is needed to help muscles recover quickly from intense exercise, and it also helps to provide a steadier flow of energy by slowing down the digestion of carbohydrate foods. Protein can come from meat, fish, eggs, dairy products, nuts, seeds, beans or lentils, depending on your dietary preferences. You'll probably also obtain some of your protein from the ingredients in recovery drinks or bars, such as whey protein powder. Healthy fats should account for around 35 per cent of your calories.

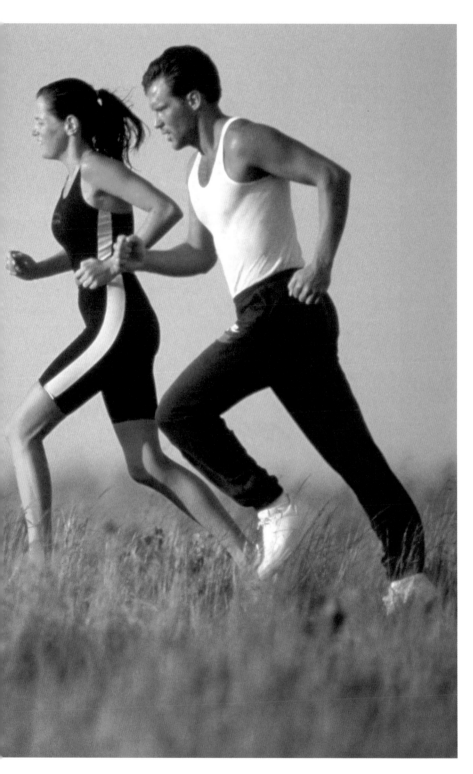

Good fats to include in your diet are oily fish, such as salmon and mackerel, avocado, olive oil, coconut oil and milk, eggs, nuts and seeds. This gives you a range of saturated, monounsaturated and polyunsaturated fats, all of which play different roles in supporting health, as well as providing energy.

On your double-run days, you'll need to plan the timing and content of your meals and snacks particularly carefully. This will give you the energy to run twice and help you to recover quickly between the sessions. Running to and from work is a common training strategy. In this case, have a quickly digested carb snack before you set off, such as a banana, white bread with honey, a fruit smoothie or some fruit juice.

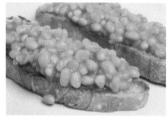

Then eat a good breakfast within 30 minutes of arriving at work, with wholegrain carbohydrate and protein. Good examples include eggs or baked beans on wholegrain toast, or porridge with added nuts and seeds. Mid-morning, have a small snack, such as a piece of fruit or 30g of mixed nuts. Eat a good-sized lunch, with a generous helping of rice, pasta or potato, plus some vegetables and protein. About 60 to 90 minutes before you run home, have an energy bar with natural ingredients (think dried fruit, nuts and seeds), a bagel with honey, or a small pasta or rice salad. Once home, eat your evening meal as soon as possible. A noodle-and-vegetable stir-fry or some simply cooked meat or fish with potatoes or

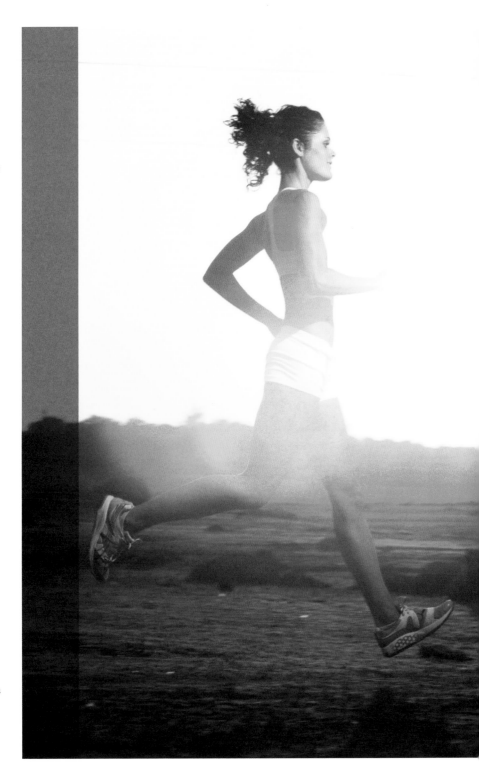

rice and veg is perfect. Try not to eat a large meal later than 8.30pm. If you have to eat late, try a smaller meal, such as a sandwich or an omelette, together with some yogurt and fruit.

If you're running for more than an hour and including higher intensity work, or for more than 90 minutes at an easy pace, you'll need to take on some carbohydrate while you train, to replenish your glycogen stores. Aim for 60g per hour. Use your long runs as an opportunity to try the sports drinks or energy gels that you plan to use during your race – check which brand will be provided. In the later stages of your run you may want to use gels that contain caffeine, to enhance performance – caffeine stimulates the nervous system. You

'Your nutritional strategy for the race itself is likely to include solid food as well as gels and sports drinks'

should also experiment with different types of solid food to see what you like and can most comfortably digest, as this will be personal to you.

It may also vary according to the temperature you are running in. In races where you'll be running for more than six hours in a single day, you're likely to want some solid food. Ideas to try in training include bananas, malt loaf, energy bars, honey sandwiches, rice pudding, rice cakes, dried fruit, pretzels (for a savoury taste and some salt) and even a baked potato. You may need to carry food with you, particularly in longer races. If you know certain foods will be available at race check

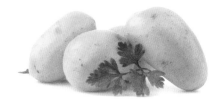

points, try these out in training. Make sure you also stay well hydrated with water, drinking according to your thirst. Remember to eat or drink some carbs and protein, such as a recovery drink or yogurt and fruit, within 20 minutes of finishing your long run.

THE WEEK BEFORE YOUR RACE

You need to make sure you start the race with your glycogen stores full, which means doing some carbohydrate loading in the last three days beforehand. It's important not to simply eat additional starchy and sugary foods on top of your normal diet; combined with the reduced running volume from your taper, this is a recipe for unwanted weight gain. Instead, gradually make carbohydrates a larger proportion of the foods you eat, and have less protein and fats. Do this by changing portion sizes (for example, two extra spoonfuls of rice, but half as much chicken). On the last day before your race, drink fruit juice and fruit smoothies between meals, as it can be hard to take on all the carbs you need through solid food. Aim for 9g to 10g of carbs per kilogram of body weight on this last day (your normal

training diet is likely to be 5g to 6g). You can use an app, such as MyFitnessPal to plan your carb load.

The night before the race, it's best to eat your evening meal no later than 7pm, depending on how early your race starts the next day. A meal high in starch but low in fat and fibre is recommended, to top up glycogen stores and help prevent race-day stomach problems. Pasta, risotto or potatoes work well, without too much veg. You should also avoid spicy food. Towards the end of your training, you should have trialled this last meal the night before a long run. If you're going to be eating in a hotel or restaurant, find out what's on the menu in advance if possible. It's not the time to be trying out new food!

RACE-DAY NUTRITION

Eat a tried-and-tested breakfast two to three hours before your race starts. White toast and honey, instant porridge and banana, an energy bar or a fruit-and-yogurt smoothie (if you can't face solid food) are good options. During the race, implement the refuelling and hydration plan you've developed during your long runs, aiming for as close to 60g of carbohydrate per hour of running as

you can tolerate. Don't forget to pack any food that you're carrying with you. Make use of the aid stations, but try to avoid eating foods you have not practised with during your long runs. Drink water according to your thirst, adding electrolyte tablets if it's a particularly hot day, to help replenish minerals lost in sweat.

RECOVERING FROM YOUR RACE

Your first priority on finishing your run is to drink or eat some easily digested carbohydrates and protein within 20 minutes, such as a specially formulated drink or bar, to start the recovery process. Then eat a full meal within two hours, including some vegetables or fruit for their antioxidant content. Tart cherry juice has been shown to help promote faster muscle recovery. You may need another snack around two hours later – this could be another bottle of recovery drink or a recovery bar. Your other priority is, clearly, rest!

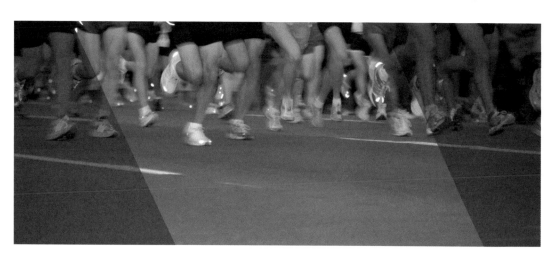

THE DEBT TO SWEAT

DON'T KNOCK PERSPIRATION. IF WE DIDN'T SWEAT WE WOULDN'T BE MUCH GOOD AT RUNNING

All runners sweat. Regardless of shape, size or fitness, sweating is part and parcel of the sport, and nothing can (or should) be done to stop it. Without sweat, runners would be in serious trouble.

It's all about thermoregulation, which is your ability to maintain a stable core body temperature. When you run you produce enough heat to put you in danger of severe overheating within ten miles. To prevent this, you sweat.

However, while sweating works very well, it comes at a price. If you don't replace the fluids you lose, you can become so dehydrated that your performance suffers – your race ends in disappointment or your long run simply ends early.

The extent to which a person sweats can vary considerably, depending on size, exercise duration and intensity, gender (men tend to sweat more than women) and the conditions – the hotter it is, the greater the sweat loss. The point at which dehydration becomes critical is widely accepted to be a loss of two per cent of body weight – *e.g* a loss of 1.4kg of weight (equal to 1.4 litres) for a 70kg runner.

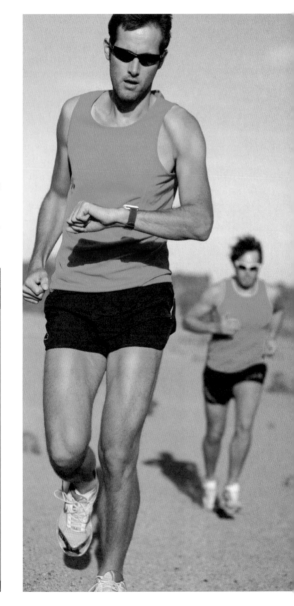

FLUID SITUATION

There is no easy answer to the question of how much you should drink, or how often, because there are so many variables. Here are some tips to keep in mind, but find out what works best for you.

▸▸ Stay comfortable by drinking according to thirst and be prudent in hot conditions – take a good mouthful every 15 minutes, for example.

▸▸ Water will do for most short runs, but for longer runs it's important to include electrolytes, particularly sodium, in your drink. Many runners report reduced incidences of cramping when they take in electrolytes, while others note improved fluid absorption or retention rates. These normally come in small sachet or tablet form and are dissolved in water. Don't forget you will also need some energy – gels are ideal.

▸▸ An isotonic sports drink provides the compromise between energy, fluid and electrolytes – perfect when training for a marathon. If an event has a designated sponsor you should try to train using that company's products.

HYDRATION NEEDS

The secret to efficient hydration is to develop good habits and to know what you need for various distances

▸▸ Stay hydrated during the day. It's amazing how many people are dehydrated when they start training, which means they risk underperforming on a long or tough training session. This one tip could make all the difference to your run.

▸▸ For a training session that lasts less than 60 minutes you probably don't need to rehydrate on the go. Sweat loss could exceed one litre, but it is unlikely fluid is required, at least from a physiological viewpoint.

▸▸ A 5K parkrun is an all-out event for many, but the duration is not long enough to require fluid intake during the race. Run hard and reward yourself with fluids afterwards.

▸▸ High-intensity (interval) session (30-60 minutes): a swig of water between reps may not assist performance but it might help you feel better and support your mental approach towards a demanding workout.

▸▸ Light-to-moderate session (60-90 minutes): some textbooks recommend drinking during such a session but see for yourself. For those preferring to run without fluids, make sure you start the session properly hydrated.

▸▸ Light-to-moderate session (more than 90 minutes): this is when you should start to develop a rehydration strategy. Water, an isotonic sports drink or a high-electrolyte solution will do the trick.

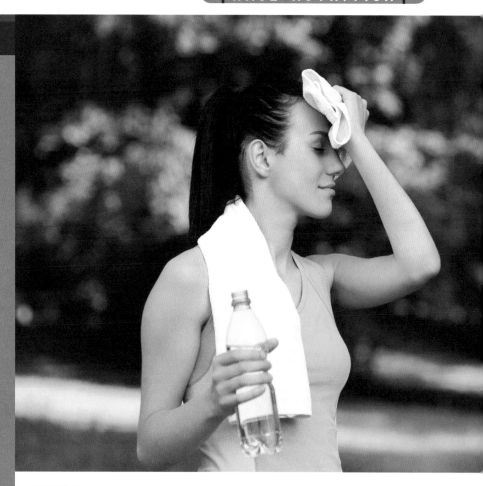

'It's amazing how many people are dehydrated when they start training'

MEASURING YOUR SWEAT RATE: THE MATHS		
Pre-exercise weight	Post-exercise weight	Fluid intake
70kg -	68.5 +	0ml
= 1.5 SWEAT LOSS (1kg lost = 1L Fluid)		

Pre-exercise weight	Post-exercise weight	Fluid intake
70kg -	68.5 +	500ml
= 2.0 SWEAT LOSS (1kg lost = 1L Fluid)		

YOU CAN MONITOR YOUR HYDRATION LEVEL USING THE PEE CHART BELOW. AIM FOR LEVELS 1 AND 2.

Target		Dehydration		Severe dehydration	
1	2	3	4	5	6

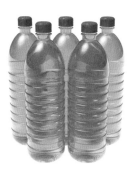

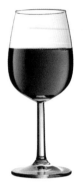

DON'T DRINK
TO YOUR HEALTH

MANY OF US LIKE A DRINK EVERY NOW AND THEN, BUT MIXING RUNNING AND ALCOHOL IS NOT A GOOD IDEA

After a hard training week or a really good race experience, you may be inclined to reward yourself with a drink or two. Yes, a couple of drinks is fine and yes, there may be a few health benefits associated with a little alcohol consumption, but as a runner there are other factors you need to consider the next time you reach for that glass of wine or pint of beer.

CALORIE CRAMMING

Alcohol is a very concentrated source of energy, with a caloric value of seven calories per gram – higher than carbohydrates and proteins (four calories per gram). If you've been watching your food intake during training, calories from alcohol can quickly add up. Alcohol is also metabolised in the body as fat – which isn't great if you're trying to trim down. Just two large glasses of red wine contain around 300 calories; to burn this off a 57kg (nine stone) woman would have to jog for at least 35 minutes.

GENDER ISSUES

Women are more susceptible than men to the effects of alcohol because of hormonal and body-fat differences. Women also tend to have less dehydrogenase, a liver enzyme that breaks down alcohol. Regular drinkers can process alcohol more easily than non-drinkers, but you need to know how alcohol affects you and your performance – preferably well before race day.

A DRINK BEFORE THE RACE?

If you like to have a drink to settle your nerves the night before a race you may wish to rethink this aspect of your pre-race ritual. While some athletes find a glass of wine can help them to relax, others find it can disturb sleep, causing blood sugar dips and nighttime waking. Alcohol is also a diuretic, so you may find you have to take more trips to the bathroom.

Alcohol is known to inhibit the metabolism of key vitamins and minerals, including B vitamins and magnesium, which are involved in energy production. Low levels of magnesium can also affect sleep and result in muscle cramps, joint aches and low energy. Avoidance is your best approach if you are not

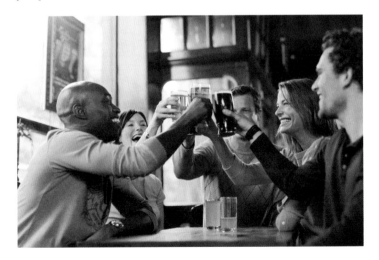

accustomed to drinking, but if you do decide to have a drink, limit yourself to one glass and have it with dinner. To combat alcohol's diuretic effect, drink 240ml of water for every alcoholic beverage you drink.

TRAINING EFFECTS

Alcohol affects the body in a wide variety of ways, many of which can have an impact on your running performance. It stimulates the heart to beat faster and widens the blood vessels (giving you that giveaway flushed complexion) but it depresses the nervous system, which can reduce exercise performance by impairing balance, coordination, visual perception and reaction time. It has also been shown to have a negative effect on strength, power and endurance.

Despite its high caloric level, alcohol is not a useful fuel source for exercise. In fact, it interferes with glucose metabolism, which can lead to an increased risk of low blood sugar, meaning fatigue will set in quicker and exercise intensity falls. If you are training hard for an endurance event, drinking alcohol on a regular basis is not going to do

anything for your performance but the odd glass is unlikely to be of great concern.

If you're doing an intensive training programme, bear in mind that alcohol can increase your risk of injuries: it can damage muscle cells, exacerbate inflammation and add to your recovery time.

Everyone metabolises alcohol differently, so always take into account the way you handle alcohol – not the more regular drinker sitting next to you. You may be wise to skip it for up to 48 hours before a long race, such as a half marathon or a marathon, to ensure enough time for proper rehydration. If you are running a shorter race and are used to the occasional glass, drink it with food and always ensure you stay hydrated before the race.

THE POST-RACE DRINK

Consuming alcohol too soon after a hard training session or race can actually impede your recovery. Alcohol is a diuretic so it increases your risk of dehydration, interferes with refuelling and impairs healing. This can leave you feeling tired, sick, and sore the next day. Drinking too

soon after a race also reduces your uptake of other carbohydrates needed to replenish your glycogen stores. It can also cause your blood sugar to rise too quickly, which may make you feel lightheaded or sick. And because alcohol dilates blood vessels it may increase inflammation, adding to the time it takes an injury to heal.

But that doesn't mean you can't enjoy a drink or two with friends (for better or for worse, it's the way many of us celebrate life's little victories). Before lifting a glass at a post-race party, have a snack high in carbs and with a little protein (a bagel with peanut butter or protein fruit smoothie) and rehydrate with 500-70ml of water or sports drink for every half a kilogram of body weight you lost while you were running.

Get in some rest and recovery time too – running the next day with a hangover is not much fun either.

'Alcohol is metabolised in the body as fat, which isn't great if you're trying to trim down'

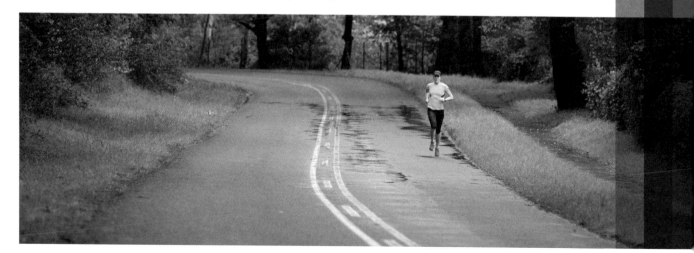

MAGNESIUM FLAIR

ARE YOU LOOKING TO BOOST YOUR PERFORMANCE, GAIN THAT COMPETITIVE EDGE AND IMPROVE YOUR RECOVERY? THEN MAKE SURE YOU'RE GETTING ENOUGH MAGNESIUM

When the subject turns to minerals (granted, this is not a common occurrence) we can usually name a few of the big hitters – calcium, iron, maybe zinc – but how many of us would leap up and shout 'Magnesium!' And even if you did, would you know what it does in the body? In short, a lot.

WHAT IS IT?

Magnesium is the fourth-most abundant mineral in the body, with approximately 60 per cent of it found in bone and 30 per cent in skeletal and cardiac muscle. Magnesium is also found in the blood and body fluids. It is involved in over 300 biochemical reactions in the body and is crucial for energy production, muscle function, protein synthesis and insulin metabolism. This makes it of critical importance for good physical performance. Yet magnesium is one of the most common nutritional deficiencies seen in athletes, resulting in reduced performance, lactic acid buildup, muscle cramping and poor recovery.

WHAT DOES IT DO?

Performance: Magnesium is vital for the conversion of glycogen to glucose – the body's main fuel during exercise.

Without sufficient levels the body switches to anaerobic metabolism, resulting in a buildup of lactic acid and associated muscle soreness and spasms. This also means if you are low in magnesium you are likely to feel tired and listless.

Magnesium also influences protein metabolism, making it important for strength and power as well as recovery. Research published in the *Journal of Nutrition* suggests that even small shortfalls in magnesium intake can seriously impair your athletic performance.

Bone Health: If you're concerned about bone health it's worth remembering that while calcium is important it does nothing without adequate levels of magnesium and vitamin D. Magnesium activates cellular enzyme activity, allowing the body to convert vitamin D into its active form to help with calcium absorption and bone building.

Recovery: Magnesium, together with calcium, is essential for optimal muscle function. A deficiency in magnesium can result in muscle and nerve twitches, spasms and cramping. Heavy exercisers often experience a buildup of lactic acid,

shin splints and painful muscles during and after exercise. Having sufficient magnesium helps speed up recovery, limit fatigue and reduce the risk of getting an injury.

Body Composition: Low levels of magnesium will decrease your insulin sensitivity, making it harder for you to lose fat. So if you are looking to change your body composition make sure you're getting enough of the stuff.

DEFICIENCY – WHY RUNNERS ARE AT RISK

Magnesium deficiency is common in runners, and people who exercise regularly are at a greater risk because of its role in energy production and metabolism. It is also lost through sweat during exercise, and in urine. Several studies, including one published in the *American Society for Clinical Nutrition*, have revealed that many athletes, particularly women, are failing to consume sufficient magnesium in their diet.

WHAT FOODS CONTAIN MAGNESIUM?

Top food sources of magnesium include unrefined wholegrains, such as wholemeal bread and wholegrain

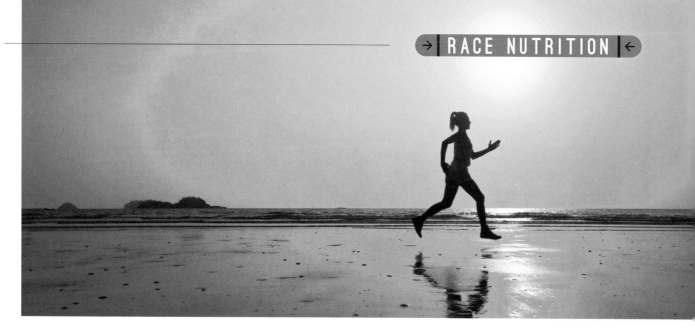

cereals, green leafy vegetables, nuts and seeds (especially pumpkin seeds), peas, beans and lentils. Some fish, such as halibut and mackerel, are also good sources. Drinking water can be an important source of magnesium, especially "hard water". But even if you have a healthy diet you may not be getting enough – you would need to eat about ten bananas to get the recommended daily amount of magnesium.

HOW MUCH DO I NEED?

The UK recommended intake for magnesium is 300mg for men and 270mg for women. The recommended intake can also be expressed in mg/kg and is roughly 6mg per kilogram of body weight. So if you weighed ten stone (63kg) this would be 378mg magnesium per day. Your daily needs may be higher if you exercise. And if you're reading this, you do.

WHAT IS THE BEST WAY TO SUPPLEMENT?

Not all forms of magnesium are created equal in terms of absorption and bioavailability (the amounts that enter the circulation and therefore have an affect on the body). You can supplement internally and externally.

Some of the best forms of supplemental magnesium are magnesium gluconate, citrate or malate, as these are readily absorbed and available to the body.

You can also increase your levels using a transdermal magnesium spray in the form of magnesium chloride. This can be applied to the skin before, during and after exercise. Because it is rapidly absorbed it makes an ideal supplement for quick results. Magnesium chloride oil or flakes can also be used as a liquid soak, either in a bath or footbath. This is ideal following exercise if you want to avoid muscle soreness and fatigue. It may also encourage a better night's sleep.

'If you are low in magnesium you are likely to feel tired and listless'

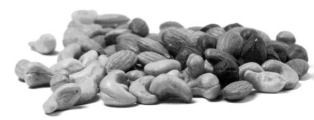

SIGNS AND SYMPTOMS OF MAGNESIUM DEFICIENCY

If you experience any of the following symptoms you may benefit from increasing your magnesium levels:

- ▸ Irregular or abnormal heartbeat
- ▸ Asthma, wheezing
- ▸ Fatigue
- ▸ Food cravings, eg carbohydrate, chocolate, salt
- ▸ Headaches and migraines
- ▸ Insomnia
- ▸ Muscle cramps and spasms
- ▸ Muscle twitches or tics
- ▸ Muscle weakness
- ▸ Numbness in hands and feet
- ▸ Aches and pains after exercise
- ▸ Poor recovery following exercise
- ▸ Low bone density, osteoporosis
- ▸ Feelings of irritability and/or lethargy
- ▸ Frequent mood swings, including depression

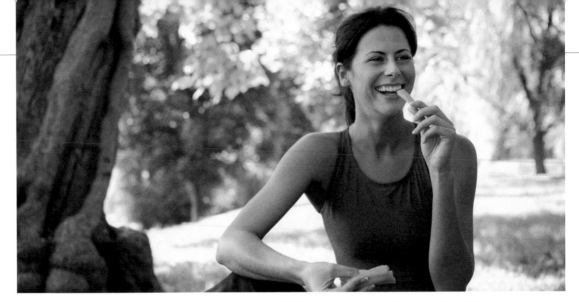

EAT WELL STAY WELL

TAKE CARE OF YOUR BODY WITH THESE NUTRITIOUS FOODS THAT WILL HELP YOU RECOVER AND REPAIR AFTER A RUN

Paying attention to your nutrition will benefit your running. It's important to eat or drink something that will give you energy before you run. But it's equally important to plan what you will eat and drink *after* a run. This is partly because you need to replace your depleted energy stores by eating foods containing carbohydrate, such as bread, cereal, vegetables and fruit. You also need to dampen down the natural inflammatory process that occurs as a result of running and help your muscles recover.

Every step you take causes microscopic damage to muscles, and wear and tear on your joints. Inflammation follows as part of the repair and adaptation process, but it should not be prolonged or it may result in injury. Certain foods have anti-inflammatory properties, so include at least one in your post-run meal or snack, which you should have within 20-45 minutes of finishing. You also need some protein to help with muscle recovery, plus some antioxidants, the plant chemicals that combat the damaging free radical chemicals generated when you exercise. Here are eight of the best foods to choose as part of your recovery meal or snack...

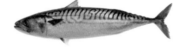

MACKEREL

This fish is a great source of omega 3 polyunsaturated fatty acids, which produce anti-inflammatory chemicals called prostaglandins. These work to dampen down the inflammatory response experienced after a hard run. Eat 100g of fresh or smoked mackerel as part of your recovery meal to obtain 2.6g of the omega 3 oils EPA and DHA. You'll also benefit from 18g of protein, to help muscle recovery, as well as some vitamin D, which also helps to reduce inflammation.

CHERRY JUICE

Cherries are rich in antioxidant chemicals called anthocyanins, which neutralise the free radical activity induced by intense exercise. Research has shown that drinking cherry juice reduces symptoms of exercise-induced muscle pain in long-distance runners. Take 30ml of cherry juice concentrate within 20 minutes of finishing your run:

'Drinking cherry juice reduces symptoms of exercise-induced muscle pain'

mix with 250ml of water or add to a smoothie. Cherry juice also contains melatonin, which may benefit your sleep, an essential part of good recovery.

PINEAPPLE

This fruit contains an enzyme called bromelain, which has been shown to have anti-inflammatory effects by decreasing production of

'Kiwi fruit contain more vitamin C than oranges'

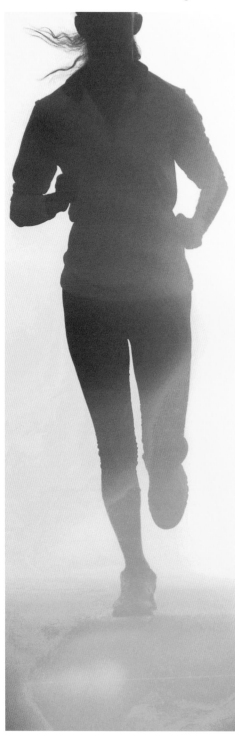

pro-inflammatory chemicals in the body. Studies have found that bromelain reduces pain and swelling, and speeds healing from injury. For a mild anti-inflammatory effect, try adding 250ml of pineapple juice to a recovery drink, or eating two to three pineapple rings as part of your post-run meal. If you are injured, a supplement containing bromelain will provide the higher amount needed.

CHICKEN

You should always include a quality source of protein in your post-run recovery meal, to help facilitate muscle repair, and you should eat it within two hours of finishing your session. Eating 100g of skinless roast chicken gives you 30g of protein, plus you get 0.7g of anti-inflammatory omega 3 fatty acids. Chicken contains more protein per gram than beef, pork, fish or egg, so it makes an excellent choice. Eat alongside vegetables or salad and some wholegrain carbohydrate.

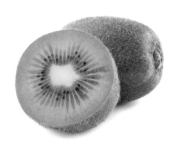

KIWI FRUIT

The connective tissues of your body, such as bones, tendons, ligaments and skin, all contain a type of protein called collagen. You need vitamin C to make collagen, so it's important to include some in your post-run meal or snack, to help repair any damage to connective tissues. It may come as a surprise but kiwi fruit contain more vitamin C than oranges. Try eating two peeled kiwi fruit or blending them into a recovery drink, for around 140mg of vitamin C.

WALNUTS

These contain more anti-inflammatory omega 3 fatty acids than any other type of nut, making walnuts a good choice of snack post-exercise or to include in your daily diet. They also contain protein, to aid muscle recovery and help keep blood vessels elastic. A 30g serving (about ten whole walnuts) provides 2.7g of omega 3 and 4.6g of protein.

RED GRAPES

These are a good source of the antioxidant quercetin, a type of plant chemical called a flavonoid, which has been shown to reduce the production of inflammatory chemicals known as TNF-alpha and interleukins. The same benefits have not been found in white grapes. After a run, eat around 15 red grapes, drink 250ml of red grape juice or add the juice to a recovery drink.

GREEN TEA

Made from unfermented tea leaves, green tea contains more antioxidants known as polyphenols than black tea. One of these polyphenols, EGCG, is thought to inhibit the expression of a gene involved in the inflammatory response. Polyphenols also neutralise the activity of damaging free radicals produced when you exercise. Drink around three cups of green tea a day, to benefit from its anti-inflammatory and antioxidant effect.

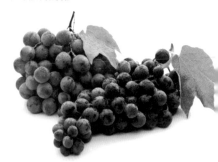

REAL-LIFE
CASE STUDIES

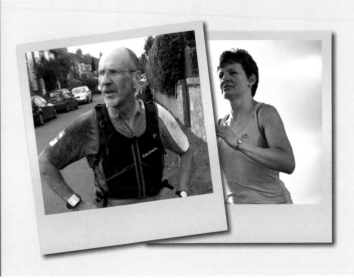

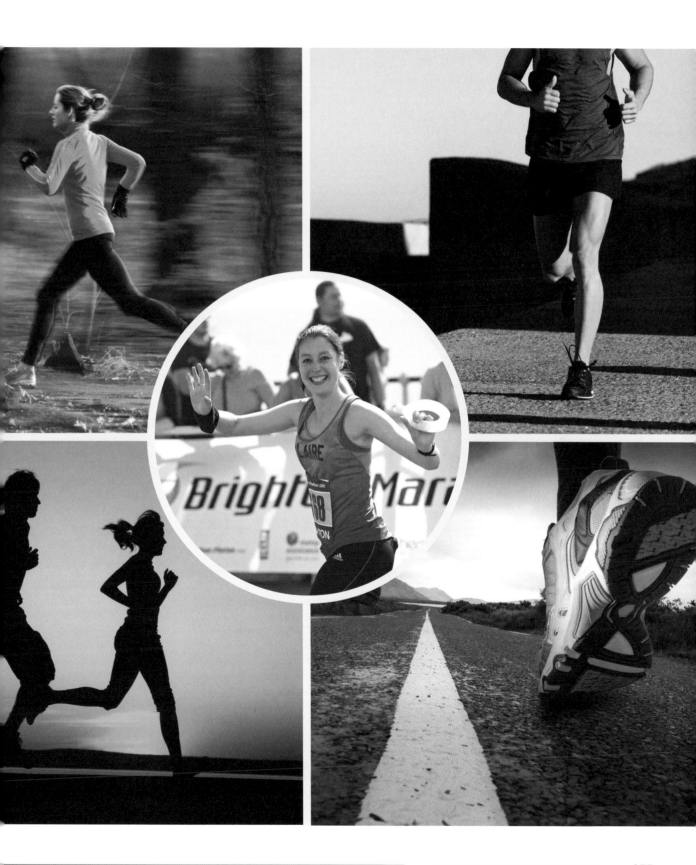

'I BECAME A BETTER RUNNER WHEN I ATE MORE'

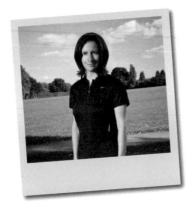

WOMEN'S RUNNING EDITOR-IN-CHIEF CHRISTINA MACDONALD STRUGGLED WITH HER RUNNING WHEN HER DIETING BECAME TOO EXTREME, AND ONLY INJURY FORCED HER TO GET THOSE BAD EATING HABITS UNDER CONTROL

Like a lot of people, I got into running for weight loss. As I built up my stamina and was able to run further, the weight began to fall off. I had never felt slimmer and fitter. But it was when I started to seriously cut back on my food intake that my problems started. I became addicted to the buzz of running, so I would take to the treadmill and run for an hour most days.

As I cut back on my food portions, the weight continued to fall off. At first, I attracted compliments from other gym goers. But after a while, the compliments stopped coming and, instead, people began to express concern. 'You're too thin,' they would say. 'You've lost too much weight.' Then the comments about my looking pale, drawn and tired started. I didn't want to hear them.

I managed to lose 18lbs (8kgs) in three months and was happy with my weight loss, but about six months later I noticed myself starting to change. My energy levels had dipped. Despite going to bed early, I couldn't seem to shift the black rings around my eyes. I was in peak condition, yet I was permanently knackered. Then my periods stopped altogether. I knew I couldn't be pregnant, it was just that I was clearly underweight for my body type.

ADDICTED TO DIETING

And yet I carried on, surviving on just 900 calories daily, and running five or six miles most days. It was ridiculous, but I couldn't seem to give up. Finally, I had to stop when I got injured. I suffered from a stress fracture that forced me to take a break from running for six weeks. You can't run on a stress fracture without doing yourself more damage (yes, I did try). During those six weeks, I managed to get my life back – I partied a bit, I caught up with friends and I started eating a bit more. It felt very good to be back in control of my life.

'Since resuming normal, healthy eating habits, my running has significantly improved'

Yes, I put a bit of weight on, but it was only half a stone (3kg) and I felt much better for it.

I learned something too… running is much more enjoyable when you have the energy to do it well. When I was dieting, I had no chance of improving as a runner. My speed and duration stayed the same and I felt awful during most of my runs.

Since resuming normal, healthy eating habits, my running has significantly improved. Yes, I've had occasional injuries, like everyone, but there's no way I'd have been able to complete five half marathons, one marathon and many 10K races without a healthy approach to food.

My favourite running foods for energy now include fruit bread, pasta, hummus and salad. And my post-run snacks include jacket potatoes, mackerel on toast with veggies or poached salmon with rice and veggies. I've never felt better – despite being 18 years older than that skinny woman who struggled on the treadmill.

Where weight loss is concerned, there simply are no short-cuts. Only a sensible training plan and a healthy approach to food will do the job.

'I BROKE THE THREE BIGGEST RACE-DAY NUTRITION RULES'

WHEN *WOMEN'S RUNNING* DEPUTY EDITOR CLAIRE CHAMBERLAIN RAN HER FIRST HALF MARATHON, A SERIES OF BAD NUTRITION DECISIONS LED TO HER BEING ALMOST UNABLE TO CROSS THE FINISH LINE

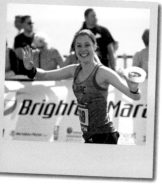

Back in 2007, I entered my first half marathon. Having run just one 5K and one 10K before, I was a relatively new runner, although my enthusiasm more than made up for this and I threw myself into training. However, there was a gaping hole in my running knowledge: I gave no thought whatsoever to race-day nutrition.

Yes, I knew I had to eat more carbs in order to have the energy to run, but for me this simply meant occasionally scoffing a flapjack on the train home from work. As far as what I should eat on race day, how much I should drink and what

gels – if any – I should try, I had no plan. And so, during the course of my first half marathon, I broke the three most important rules of race-day nutrition. The result? I collapsed by the side of the road, needed first aid and limped to the finish line in a delirious state. The rules I broke were these...

'I kept gulping water to stave off dehydration, little knowing I was slowly diluting my blood sodium levels'

RULE ONE: EAT A TRIED AND TESTED RACE-DAY BREAKFAST

Any experienced runner knows to eat a carb-based breakfast the morning of a race. Nothing new, nothing fancy, just something you know your stomach will

tolerate. During training, I was used to eating porridge in the mornings. However, I was so nervous on the morning of the half marathon I could hardly touch it. I felt sick with the anticipation of the 13.1 miles that lay ahead and consequently ate less than half my normal amount, meaning I turned up to the start line under-fuelled. Oops. Not good.

RULE TWO: DON'T OVER-DRINK

As I said, I'd only ever taken part in a 5K and 10K. At the 5K there were no drinks stations. At the 10K there was one. Over the course of this half marathon, I was encountering a drinks station every few miles. As it was a hot day, I figured the best thing I could do was take a drink at every water station (I now cringe at this). I'd never heard of hyponatraemia before. Needless to say, I have now. I kept gulping water to stave off dehydration, little knowing I was slowly diluting my blood sodium levels. Which is why, at around mile 12,

things started getting hazy. I stopped in the middle of the pack and swayed unsteadily. A lovely runner grabbed my arm and ushered me to the pavement, where race marshals sat me down. Which was lucky, as I promptly blacked out.

When I came round, I couldn't remember my name, had a strong desire to take my shoes and socks off, and was mumbling jargon to everyone. Evidently not my finest hour... but things were about to get worse. A friendly runner stopped to see if I was all right and very kindly gave me one of his energy gels. Which leads me to rule three...

RULE THREE: NEVER TRY GELS YOU HAVEN'T PRACTISED USING IN TRAINING

Deciding energy was exactly what I needed, I downed the energy gel in several gulps... only to throw it all back up seconds later. Not quite the boost I was looking for.

After half an hour recuperating by the roadside, I did manage to get to my feet and walk the half mile to the finish line. And while the race is one of my more memorable half marathons for all the wrong reasons, on the plus side I now have three of the most important race-day nutrition rules drummed into my brain. Six years and many half marathons and marathons later, I've never made the same mistakes again.

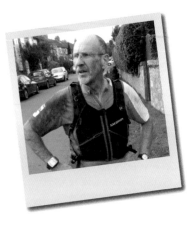

'I WAS TIRED ALL THE TIME'

SEASONED RUNNER GARY TEBBUTT WAS LOW ON ENERGY AND SUFFERING DURING HIS LONG RUNS, UNTIL HE OVERHAULED HIS FUELLING STRATEGY

In summer 2012, I joined *Men's Running* magazine's Operation Ultra project to train for an ultra marathon. As a seasoned marathon runner, I wanted a new challenge and this was a chance to get world class support to do so.

At the start of the training programme, I sat down with *Men's Running* coach Nick Anderson to go through my running history. I told him I thought I was doing too much running because I was tired all the time. At this point he stopped me and asked about my diet.

DODGY DIETING

I've battled with my weight all my life and have always counted the calories daily. I broke down what I ate for Nick. I was consuming 1,750 calories a day, adding 100 calories per mile on run days, but the weight was still going on. I would often skip breakfast on non-run days, then have fruit for the rest of the day, maybe a salad for lunch, and finish with a sensible dinner of meat and vegetables.

At weekends I binged on biscuits and sweet things, but come Monday, I was back on the diet. It was a dieting roller-coaster all the time.

Nick explained that, having done this for months, my body had gone into starvation mode and my metabolism had slowed down. He tried to convince me I needed to eat more to lose weight. I knew I needed to fuel my ultra training, but as I already felt overweight, I was worried. However, I gave it a go.

Within days I felt different – my energy levels were up. My general eating was better. I had more substantial breakfasts of wholemeal bread and peanut butter, cereal or porridge. I snacked on oatcakes and rice cakes, and sipped on sports drinks. I had bigger lunches, with pasta and rice, and I stopped counting calories.

QUALITY TRAINING

Since adopting this new nutrition strategy, my weight has become much more stable, but the biggest difference I noticed was at the start of my

long runs. Previously, in the first four miles, I felt tight, stiff and my heart rate would race, even at ten or 11 minute-mile pace. Then I would settle down and get into my run. Since I started eating well and fuelling properly, I rarely get that. I can head out of the door and feel normal from mile one.

During my long runs, I also used to consume the bare

'Since I started eating well and fuelling properly, I can head out of the door and feel normal from mile one'

minimum of energy gels or drinks, to ensure maximum calorie burn. I'd get through the runs, but come Monday and Tuesday I was too tired to do any quality training sessions. Now, by eating during long runs and fuelling properly, I finish much fresher and the following day I can get straight back into it, so the quality of my sessions has improved too. I would also always have an easy day before

a long run, but with my new nutrition strategy, I'm able to do a 75-minute hill session on the Saturday and a 20-miler on Sunday morning, then go out again that night. To do that on my old diet would have been impossible.

I used to be full of trepidation on my long runs, thinking 'Oh God, I've got to run for three hours'. Now I look forward to

running because I'm fuelled up and I know I'm not going to suffer in the first few miles. To sum up my new philosophy, it's 'Eat to run, don't run to eat'.

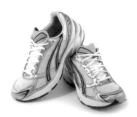

'I'VE LEARNED TO EAT ON THE RUN'

BUSY MUM AND ULTRA RUNNER ANNE-MARIE LATEGAN HAS SOME VERY SIMPLE RULES WHEN IT COMES TO NUTRITION FOR LONG-DISTANCE RUNNING. AND SHE STICKS TO THEM

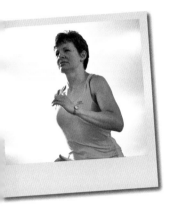

Ultra running has become part of my lifestyle. I don't change my diet in the few days before a race because I would not do that during my training. I never run on an empty stomach and have three breakfasts that I can choose from, depending on the type of race I'm preparing for and when it starts. If it's a noon start, which is typical for a 24-hour race, I will have scrambled eggs on wholemeal or brown toast. For earlier race starts I will either have a wrap with peanut butter, or muesli mixed with hemp protein and soya yogurt.

I eat three meals a day and one snack mid-morning. Since I starting ultra running I haven't increased the volume of food that I eat. The hardest thing to get used to is eating on the run. During an ultra event I normally get through two or three meals – I prefer to get some substantial food while I run. I have experimented with a lot of different foods, supplements, electrolytes and gels. Some caused severe stomach cramps;

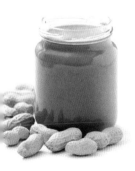

others have worked much better. The most important thing I have learned is that the more natural the food is, the better my stomach can cope with it.

When I go out for a long training run or line up for a race, I will have natural, cold-pressed fruit bars and protein bars because there are no chemical processes involved in their production. My body is not designed to break down chemicals, so if I'm already pushing it to the limit during the run I don't want to make it work harder by giving it unknown chemicals that it doesn't know how to digest.

CHEMICAL-FREE

My preferred protein is hemp. Again, there is no chemical process involved in making it. This type of protein has very high levels of branch-chain amino acids (BCAAs). These contain three types of amino acids (the building blocks of protein) that help to make different proteins within your muscles. They help you to

generate more energy, limit fatigue and speed up your recovery. I also supplement with extra BCAAs before, during and after a run.

WRAPPED UP

During long runs I always have peanut butter wraps. They are a good source of slow-release energy and they're easily digestible. My hydration is determined by the distance and the weather conditions. I will always drink water and have a

'The most important thing I have learned is that the more natural the food is, the better my stomach can cope with it'

variety of other drinks to prevent boredom.

The first is a 50:50 blend of Coca-Cola and water. I also have two types of electrolytes. One is high in calories, which helps to reduce the amount of solid food I need to eat when I'm replacing lost electrolytes. The other type contains hardly any calories but it does contain caffeine. I like to use caffeine because it helps me to focus, especially during the later stages of the race and especially at night.

EASY NUTRITION FOR RUNNERS

NUTRITION FOR HEALTH & RECOVERY

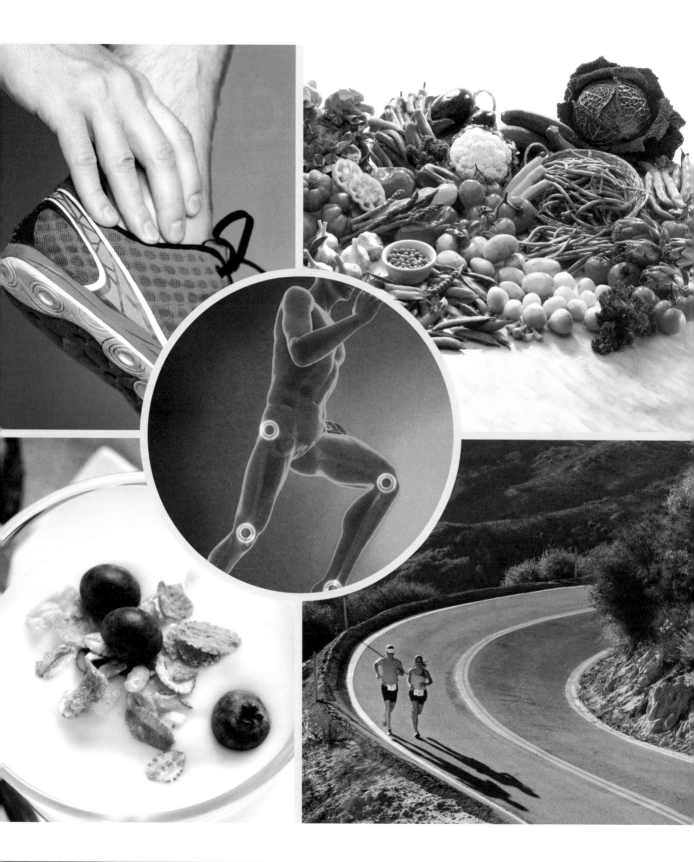

SNACK ATTACK

NEED A SNACK BEFORE YOUR RUN? IT'S TIME TO DITCH THOSE SUGAR-FILLED FOODS AND INTRODUCE SOME HEALTHY OPTIONS TO FUEL YOUR BODY

As a runner, eating a nutrient-rich, energy-boosting snack before a run is an important fuelling strategy. The trouble is knowing what and how much to eat. This will, of course, partly depend on how long you are running for and the time of day, but there are some general principles that should be kept in mind.

Most runners find they perform best on a carbohydrate-

'View snacks as a means not just to fuel your run, but also to provide you with additional nutrients'

based snack that's low in fibre. Including some protein and healthy fats can help balance blood sugar during a long run, but too much can lead to digestive upset, as these foods break down more slowly in the digestive tract.

However, don't be tempted to grab a bag of sweets or a cake on the way home from work. These high-calorie, nutrient-poor options will do little to nourish your body with the

vitamins and minerals it needs for energy production. Instead, view snacks as a means not just to fuel your run, but also to provide you with additional nutrients not provided by your meals. To curb pre-run hunger, aim to eat 15-60 minutes before running. Keep the portion small – you are looking for 200-300 calories. However, if you're planning to do a long running session, you may need to eat something more substantial about two hours beforehand.

Here are some great healthy options to provide the fuel your body needs…

THE ULTRA SHAKE

Can't face food before a run? Try Metagenics Ultra Meal Vanilla or Chocolate blended with a banana and coconut water. It combines slow- and quick-release carbohydrates, electrolytes and protein with vitamins and minerals for energy production.

297 calories
18g protein
51.2g carbohydrate
2.2g fat

YOGURT CRUNCH

Fat-free Greek yogurt is easy to digest and full of healthy probiotic bacteria. It's also a

good source of protein and calcium. Spoon 125g into a bowl and top with a handful of toasted oats and seeds, plus a handful of berries (30g) for a hefty hit of anti-inflammatory antioxidants.

216 calories
18.8g protein
17.4g carbohydrate
7.8g fat

FROZEN BANANA AND GREEN TEA ICE CREAM

Slice four bananas and place them in the freezer for two to three hours. Once they're frozen, place in a high-speed blender or food processor with 1tsp Matcha green tea powder and a dash of milk or milk alternative, and blend to form instant ice cream (serves two). It's high in carbohydrates and vitamin B6 for energy production, plus the green tea contains plenty of antioxidants to counter muscle soreness and inflammation. For a longer run, you could add a scoop of protein powder to the mixture, to help keep blood sugar balanced.

199 calories
5.1g protein
43.2g carbohydrate
0.7g fat

HEALTHY ENERGY BAR

Nakd bars are a great light option, combining nuts and dried fruits. This is perfect 30-60 minutes before a short run to perk up energy levels. For something more substantial, try a TREK Energy Bar, which contains slow-releasing oats, ginseng and gingko to increase energy levels.

Nakd Coca Orange Bar:

145 calories
4g protein
16g carbohydrate
7g fat

TREK Energy Bar Berry:

204 calories
11g protein
38g carbohydrate
2g fat

MACA CHOCOLATE SMOOTHIE

Maca is a Peruvian herb known to help the body cope with stress, making it a popular choice with athletes. Blend a tablespoon with 500ml Chocolate Rice Dream, one banana and 1tbsp cashew nut butter (serves two). This is a terrific combination of easy-to-digest carbs, protein and a little healthy fat (from the cashew nut butter). It's a

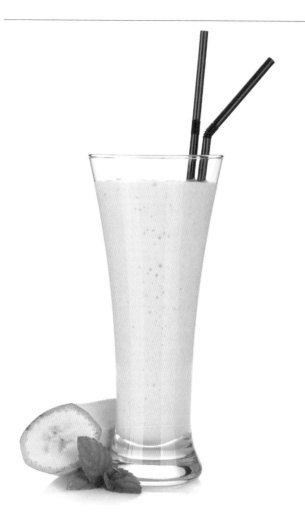

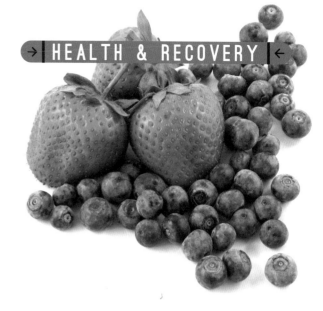

great choice 30-60 minutes before a run.

265 calories
4.6g protein
47.2g carbohydrate
6.4g fat

PORRIDGE WITH RAISINS AND CINNAMON

If bread and bagels bloat you out, try gluten-free oats. They're a great source of slow-release carbohydrate and the addition of raisins gives you some instant carbs to kick-start your run. Aim to eat one to two hours before running. Cinnamon is also a useful spice, shown to improve insulin function, which balances blood sugars. Make with 40g oats, semi-skimmed milk and water, 1tbsp raisins and 1tsp cinnamon.

298 calories
10.1g protein
50.7g carbohydrate
5.9g fat

RICE CAKES WITH DRIED APRICOTS AND ALMOND NUT BUTTER

Rice cakes are easy on the stomach, and low in calories and fibre, yet will provide you with enough calories to sustain a run. Dried apricots are a good source of iron. Add some almond nut butter to provide protein to balance your blood sugar. Try two rice cakes with 1tbsp nut butter and three to four dried apricots.

219 calories
7.5g protein
21.6g carbohydrate
11.4g fat

APPLE SLICES AND PEANUT BUTTER

Cut up an apple and top the slices with wholegrain peanut butter. Apples are a good source of quercetin, an antioxidant that helps counter inflammation, while peanuts provide protein and healthy fats for sustained energy. Accompany with a glass of coconut water to quickly hydrate and balance electrolytes.

216 calories
7.2g protein
21.7g carbohydrate
11.2g fat

WHY SNACK?

Eating a nutrient-rich snack provides your body with additional glycogen, to help fuel your run. But it also helps stabilise your blood sugar, to keep you energised and motivated. Low levels of stored glycogen will make your run hard work and you'll tire more quickly. It will also cause your adrenals to kick in, producing cortisol to help break down stored glycogen. This can put additional strain on your body and deplete key nutrients, such as vitamin C, magnesium and B vitamins – all of which are important for energy production. In addition, by taking the edge off your appetite, you are less likely to overeat later!

MORE MILES = MORE FOOD

UPPING YOUR MILEAGE WITHOUT INCREASING YOUR FOOD INTAKE COULD SERIOUSLY HINDER YOUR PERFORMANCE. HERE'S WHAT YOU SHOULD BE EATING TO FUEL YOUR LONG-DISTANCE RUNS

Whether you're building up to a marathon, a half marathon or even a 10K, upping your weekly training mileage means upgrading your diet too. Don't make the mistake of thinking extra mileage is a great way to burn off the pounds. While you may lose weight initially, intense training without adequate calories and nutrients can quickly result in overtraining syndrome, the symptoms of which include decreased performance, fatigue, loss of motivation, depression and an increased chance of illness.

Intense training demands good nutrition. Rule number one – if you want to have enough energy to complete your new, tougher workouts, you will have to eat more food. While this isn't a licence to eat whatever you want, you must match your calories to your training volume. Failing to eat enough calories, carbohydrate and dietary fat when you step up your training volume is one of the most common reasons for low energy levels in runners. Under-eating coupled with intense training leads to low glycogen stores and increased levels of stress hormones, such as adrenaline and cortisol, which, in turn, inhibit the immune system. So you could quickly end up feeling run-down and more susceptible to colds and infections.

COUNTING THE CALORIES

A good rule of thumb is to multiply your mileage by 100 (running burns approximately 100 calories per mile). So, a five-mile run will burn roughly 500 calories, irrespective of your speed. To get a more accurate estimate of calories burned, multiply your weight (in pounds) by 0.72. So, a 54kg (119lb) runner will burn 86 calories per mile, while a 67kg (148lb) runner will burn 106 calories per mile.

If you increase your weekly mileage by ten miles, you will need to eat an extra 1,000 calories a week – that's 143 calories a day – to maintain your muscle glycogen stores and prevent a rise in cortisol. Fail to adjust your calorie intake and you risk a drop in energy, slower times, inability to complete training runs and, over time, a loss of muscle tissue. It's like expecting your car to travel 50 miles but only providing enough fuel for it to travel 20 miles; you're going to stop before you finish and you won't be able to get going again.

CRUCIAL CARBOHYDRATE

Some runners seem to have a carbohydrate phobia, owing to the misguided belief that carbohydrate is responsible for weight gain. But it

has long been established that adequate carbohydrate intake is needed to maintain muscle glycogen levels during intense training. This is critical for sustaining high training volumes, because muscle glycogen is the main fuel stored in muscles that's used during endurance training and racing.

A study at the University of Birmingham found that runners consuming a relatively low carbohydrate intake (5.4g/kg body weight/day) during 11 days of intense training experienced a drop in their running performance, a significant worsening of their mood, fatigue and muscle soreness. These symptoms were reversed when the runners then performed the same training regime with a higher carbohydrate intake (8.5g/kg body weight/day).

HOW MUCH IS ENOUGH?

During periods of moderate-intensity training, most runners will need between 5g and 7g of carbohydrate per kilogram of body weight per day. But during more intense training periods, with training runs of two hours or more, they will need to increase that daily carbohydrate intake to between 7g and 10g per kilogram of body weight per day. So, a 60kg (132lb) runner training one

CARBOHYDRATE NEEDS FOR RUNNING				
Number of hours' exercise per day	Carbohydrate/ kg body weight/day	Carbohydrate/ day for a 50kg person	Carbohydrate/ day for a 60kg person	Carbohydrate/ day for a 70kg person
0–1 hour	5–6g	250–300g	300–360g	350–420g
1–2 hours	6–7g	300–350g	360–420g	420–490g
3–4 hours	7–8g	350–400g	420–480g	490–560g
More than 4 hours	8–10g	400–500g	480–600g	560–700g

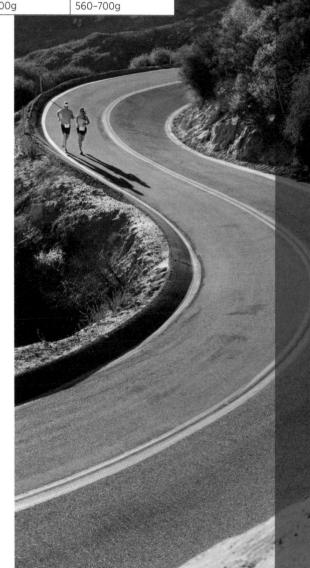

to two hours each day would need 300–420g of carbohydrate daily; but 420–600g daily if training for two hours or longer.

PUTTING IT INTO PRACTICE

For an idea of how much food you need to eat, the menu below contains approximately 400g of carbohydrate, which is enough to fuel around two hours of daily exercise for a runner weighing 60kg (132lb):

MENU

Breakfast: 2 slices of toast with margarine and honey; 2 bananas

Lunch: 1 large baked potato (200g) with margarine, half a tin (200g) of baked beans, and 2 tablespoons (40g) grated cheese; salad; 1 fruit yogurt

Dinner: Large bowl of pasta (125g dried weight); chicken (125g) or cheese (40g); vegetables

Snacks : 2 pieces of fresh fruit; 400ml fruit juice; 2 cereal bars; 1 fruit yogurt

Total energy = 2,800 calories
Total carbohydrate = 411g

GETTING THE BALANCE RIGHT

As a rough guide, if you're struggling to recover fully between training sessions and frequently lack energy while training, then you may not be eating enough and could be at risk of overtraining. This could lead to a number of problems, including:

▸▸ Lack of progress (in fact, your training may regress).
▸▸ Increased risk of injury.
▸▸ Frequent minor illnesses (owing to a weakened immune system).
▸▸ Poor performance in races.

On the other hand, if you're putting on unwanted pounds, cutting back on energy-dense foods that are high in fat and sugar (such as crisps, confectionery and sugary drinks) will help you attain a healthier weight. You'll feel better too.

TIMING IS EVERYTHING

Consuming adequate carbohydrate is particularly important in the period immediately following intense exercise, as this can boost recovery, help prevent overtraining and allow you to get the most out of your runs.

High carbohydrate foods should be the mainstay of your meals before and after your long runs. Aim for around 200g of carbohydrate two to four hours before a long run. If you run first thing in the morning, eat plenty of high carbohydrate foods at your evening meal and then have a sports drink, diluted fruit juice (50:50 juice and water) or squash (diluted 1:6 with water) before heading out for your morning run. If you need a snack half an hour before a run, aim for 30-60g of carbohydrate (for example, two bananas or two cereal bars).

During your run, consume 30-60g of carbohydrate per hour (for example, 500ml of an isotonic sports drink or one to two energy gels) if you're exercising for longer than an hour.

Adding protein to your post-run recovery drinks and meals can have further benefits. After your long run, drink 500ml of flavoured milk or eat a banana and drink 500ml of skimmed milk, as this protein-carbohydrate combination will accelerate muscle recovery.

In short, nutrition plays a critical role in supporting intense training. As you step up your mileage, you must step up your food intake, so increase your carbohydrate and protein intake, plan your daily eating strategy and include a post-run recovery meal that contains both carbohydrate and protein. Bon appétit!

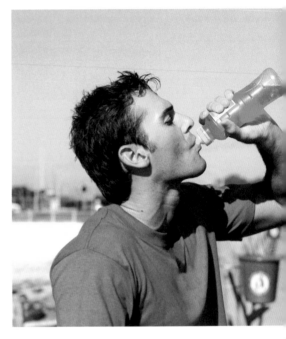

'If you want to have enough energy to complete your new, tougher workouts, you will have to eat more food'

ARE YOU OVERTRAINING?

If you're not consuming enough calories and nutrients to support your training, you may suffer from the following:

▸▸ **An increase in resting heart rate of around ten per cent (about five beats per minute above your normal rate).**

▸▸ Reaching training heart rate zone much sooner into a run than usual.

▸▸ **Increased time for heart rate to recover between intervals.**

▸▸ Inability to make progress in fitness goals.

▸▸ **Extreme fatigue.**

▸▸ Depression or lack of enthusiasm for training.

▸▸ **Regular injuries (such as sprains and strains), colds or upper respiratory tract infections.**

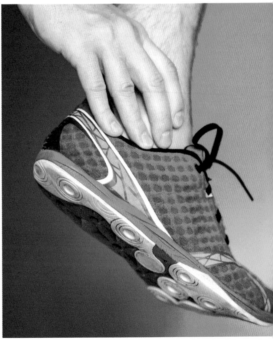

If you love this, try *Men's Running* or *Women's Running*

Order your FREE copy today

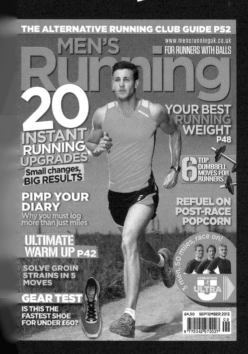

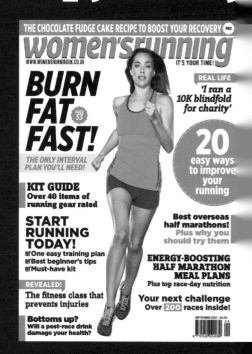

The UK's first running magazine just for men.

Whether it's racing, losing weight, getting fit, looking for new gear and gadgets or reading the most eye-popping, inspirational stories from the world of running, we take pride in offering you all this and more in the only magazine dedicated to running men everywhere.

The UK's first running magazine just for women

Ideal for beginners and regular runners. Includes features on getting started, improving your running and boosting stamina plus training plans for a variety of distances and abilities. Each issue includes weight-loss, gym training, health, nutrition and inspirational real-life stories.

How to get your FREE copy

Try *Men's Running* totally FREE.

Text **'Runner'** to **60300** to claim your FREE issue today

Or call **0845 286 3067** & quote **'Runner'**

Try *Women's Running* totally FREE.

Text **'Runner'** to **60300** to claim your FREE issue today

Or call **0845 286 3067** & quote **'Runner'**

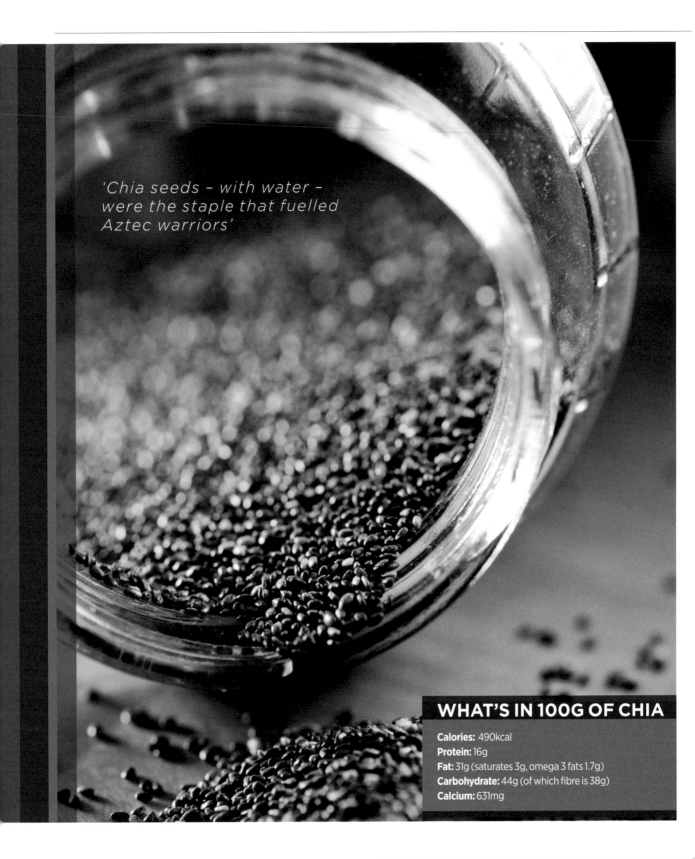

'Chia seeds – with water – were the staple that fuelled Aztec warriors'

WHAT'S IN 100G OF CHIA

Calories: 490kcal
Protein: 16g
Fat: 31g (saturates 3g, omega 3 fats 1.7g)
Carbohydrate: 44g (of which fibre is 38g)
Calcium: 631mg

THE RUNNING FOOD

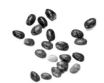

OMEGA 3 FATS ARE A RUNNER'S NATURAL RECOVERY AID. THE BEST SOURCES ARE OILY FISH BUT VEGETARIANS CAN GET THEIR OMEGA BOOST FROM CHIA SEEDS TO MAINTAIN GOOD HEALTH AND TOP PERFORMANCE

WHAT ARE OMEGA 3 FATS ?

Omega 3s are one of the key nutrients all runners should include in their diet. Our bodies produce inflammatory chemicals, either through running or other forms of stress, trauma or injury. Omega 3 fats help counter that inflammation by producing natural anti-inflammatory compounds called prostaglandins. By reducing inflammation you can help your body heal and recover faster, as well as reduce post-exercise muscle soreness.

WHAT ELSE?

Research has shown that omega 3s may help prevent exercise-induced asthma, improving post-exercise lung function and supporting heart health. They are also vital for keeping our body's cell membranes flexible and healthy; this is important for cell communication of hormones and neurotransmitters, which influences our mood and cognitive function.

They are also involved in fat metabolism, so by optimising your omega intake you can help keep your body composition healthy, promoting fat burning rather than fat storage.

WHERE CAN WE GET THEM?

Omega 3 fats are termed "essential" because they cannot be manufactured by the body – they have to be obtained from our diet. However, one of the problems with our Western diet is that it is relatively high in omega 6 fats (found in many vegetable oils, nuts, seeds and processed foods) but low in omega 3 fats. Traditionally, our diet had a more balanced intake. Today, it is estimated our intake is between 10:1 to 20:1 of omega 6 to omega 3 fats.

Studies have demonstrated that this high intake of omega 6 compared with omega 3 fats has shifted our physiologic state to one that is pro-inflammatory, which has led to an increase in inflammation-related conditions, which range from heart disease to psoriasis. In fact, recent research from the Harvard School of Public Health found that higher blood levels of omega 3 could reduce the chances of dying from heart disease by more than a third.

The main animal sources of omega 3 fats (Docosahexaenoic acid or DHA, and Eicos-apentaenoic acid or EPA) are oily fish such as sardines, salmon, herring and fresh tuna. Canned tuna is not a good source because omega 3 levels are reduced in the sourcing and canning process. Fish higher in the food chain can contain high levels of mercury, so you should restrict your intake of larger fish such as tuna and swordfish (the Food Standards Agency recommends that people eat at least two portions of fish a week, one of which should be oily).

WHAT ABOUT VEGETARIANS?

Vegetarian sources of omega 3 fatty acids, known as alpha-linolenic acid (ALA), are found in a range of foods, including flaxseed, hemp seeds, chia seeds, walnuts, pumpkin seeds, soybeans and green leafy vegetables. This type of omega 3 fat needs to be converted by the body into the longer chain fats found in animal sources, but research suggests this conversion is relatively inefficient. So if you are a vegetarian, aim to consume these foods every day and consider taking a vegetarian DHA supplement.

WHAT ABOUT THESE CHIA SEEDS?

One of the best plant sources of omega 3s are chia seeds, with 30 per cent of their fat coming from omega 3 and ten per cent from omega 6. Chia, or salvia hispanica L, is a member of the mint family and is native to Mexico and South America; it has been enjoyed for centuries as a food and medicine. Known as "the running food", chia seeds – with water – were the staple that fuelled Aztec warriors.

Not only are they rich in omega 3s, but chia seeds also pack a serious nutritional punch for runners, being high in antioxidants, vitamins, minerals, fibre and protein. Just 28g of the seeds contain nearly 20 per cent of your daily calcium needs, as well as 4g protein and 11g fibre. Chia seeds are incredibly rich in soluble fibre and when they are soaked with water they form a gel. The gel can then be added to drinks or dishes to slow down the rate of digestion. This makes it the perfect fuel for long runs. As chia seeds hold ten times their weight in water, they are a great hydrator too. Chia seeds can be added to smoothies, protein shakes and a range of sweet and savoury dishes.

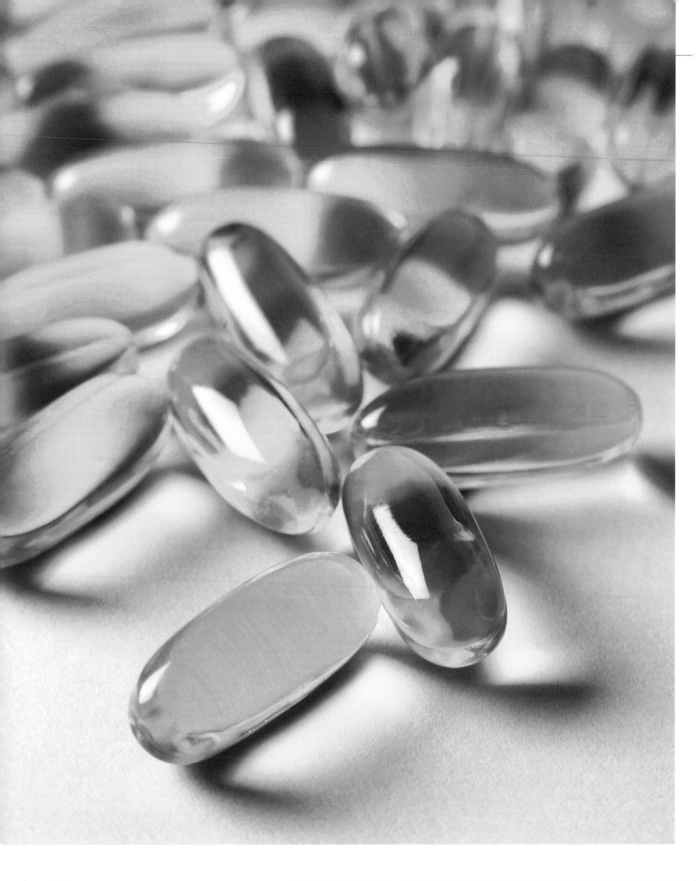

FISH OILS – IS THERE ANYTHING THEY CAN'T DO?

YOU KNOW THEY ARE GOOD FOR YOUR BRAIN AND YOUR HEART, BUT DID YOU KNOW FISH OILS CAN HELP YOUR RUNNING TOO?

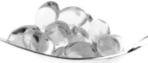

More and more runners are taking an interest in the power of fish oils. Although they've long been associated with heart health and brain development, new research links the anti-inflammatory properties of these oils to numerous benefits for runners – from the enhancement of aerobic capacity to the relief of post-run joint pain.

Oily fish are an excellent source of omega 3 fats, a group of unsaturated fats that are vital to health. Sources include mackerel, sardines, herring, trout, pilchards and salmon. Fresh tuna is an oily fish but canned doesn't count as oily because much of the oil is removed during the canning process. The Food Standards Agency recommends eating two portions of fish a week, one of which should be oily. A portion is 140g, roughly six pilchards or a medium salmon steak. The minimum requirement for omega 3s is 0.9g a day, which you can get from one portion

(140g) of oily fish a week or one tablespoon of an omega 3-rich oil daily (see table 'the omega 3 content of various foods').

There are three main types of omega 3s: the short-chain fatty acid, alpha linolenic acid (ALA, found in plant sources), and the long-chain fatty acids, eicosapentanoic acid (EPA) and docosahexanoic acid (DHA), both found only in fish oils.

Including omega 3s in your diet may be a good way of boosting your aerobic fitness and improving your race times. According to research at the University of California, US, supplementation with omega 3s for six weeks increases blood flow and oxygen delivery to the muscles during exercise, and decreases resting blood pressure (1, 2). The extra oxygen may raise maximal oxygen consumption (VO2 max). And in a study carried out at Western Washington University, people who supplemented their diet with fish oil supplements (4g of omega 3s per day) for 10 weeks

How can vegetarians get enough omega 3s?

If you're a vegetarian, it's more difficult to get your omega 3 quota because the most abundant source is oily fish. In fact, fish is the only source of the long-chain omega 3 fatty acids, eicosapentanoic acid (EPA) and docosahexanoic acid (DHA).

But you can also get omega 3s from nuts and seeds, in the form of alpha-linolenic acid (ALA). The body will convert this ALA into EPA and DPA. Unfortunately, as this conversion process isn't all that efficient, you'll need to eat quite a lot of ALA to produce levels of EPA and DHA comparable to those that can be obtained by eating fish.

To compensate for this, the Vegetarian Society recommends 4g ALA a day, equivalent to a couple of handfuls (50g) of walnuts or two teaspoons of flaxseed oil. A daily portion of green veg will also add useful amounts.

while following a moderate exercise programme, increased their aerobic fitness by 11 per cent, compared with controls who did not take supplements.

POST-RUN BENEFITS

Feeling sore after your run? Well, adding omega 3s to your diet may make you hurt less and heal faster too. Strenuous running causes the body to produce inflammatory substances that are responsible for delayed-onset muscle soreness. A 2009 study published in the *Clinical Journal of Sports Medicine* found that people who took a fish oil supplement for 30 days had significantly less muscle soreness and inflammation 48 hours after intense exercise.

Taking omega 3s may also help you run longer before fatigue sets in. A US study in the *European Journal of Applied Physiology* found a trend towards increased time before fatigue in those who took a daily omega 3 supplement for four weeks.

'Omega 3 increases blood flow and oxygen delivery to the muscles during exercise'

And omega 3s may be good news for those who are prone to exercise-induced asthma. Strenuous exercise can sometimes trigger a narrowing of the airways, restricting airflow. In studies from Indiana University, three weeks of fish oil supplementation significantly improved exercise asthma symptoms in athletes, reduced airway inflammation and improved lung function.

WEIGHT-LOSS

If you're running to shift excess pounds, adding omega 3s to your diet may help you achieve your goal faster. Researchers at the University of South Australia found that overweight women who undertook a moderate walk/run exercise programme three times a week while taking fish oil supplements lost an average of 2kg over three months while eating whatever they wanted. In contrast, those who exercised but did not take the supplements did not lose any weight; nor did those who took supplements but did not exercise. Researchers concluded that combining fish oil supplementation with regular aerobic exercise increases the body's fat-burning ability by improving the flow of blood to the muscles during exercise.

While there's no proof that exercise or running causes joint problems, such as rheumatoid arthritis, those with achy knees will be pleased to learn that omega 3s may bring relief. Trials at the University of Pittsburgh Medical Centre report improvements in morning stiffness and joint tenderness with the regular intake of fish oil supplements for up to three months. In fact, researchers have found that omega 3s are as effective as prescriptive medication, such as ibuprofen, at easing joint pain.

After one month of taking supplements, 60 per cent stated that their joint pain had improved. In 2007, a review of 17 studies by Canadian researchers added weight to these findings and concluded that omega 3s effectively reduce joint pain intensity and the number of tender joints. There's no special diet or miracle food that cures joint pain, but it may be helped by increasing your intake of omega 3s. Opt for a supplement containing 200-400mg omega 3s per capsule. Take one capsule before meals two or three times a day.

CAN YOU EAT TOO MUCH OILY FISH?

The FSA warns against eating too much oily fish because of the risk of consuming pollutants, such as mercury and polychlorinated biphenyls (PCBs), which can build up in the body. At high levels, mercury can cause symptoms of toxicity including depression, memory loss and fatigue. PCBs, which may increase cancer risk, have been banned since 1976 but still show up at low levels in some oily fish. Women who are pregnant, breastfeeding or planning to become pregnant are advised not to eat more than two weekly portions (as mercury can be harmful to the developing brain) and completely avoid high-mercury fish such as shark, swordfish and marlin. Those who won't have a baby in the future (as well as men) may eat up to four portions a week.

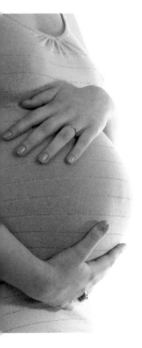

FISH OIL SUPPLEMENTS AND PREGNANCY

There are two types of supplements: those made from the fish liver (such as cod liver oil) and those made from the fish body. If you're pregnant, avoid fish liver oil supplements, because they contain high levels of vitamin A, which may harm your unborn baby. Fish oils not derived from the liver (the label will tell you) are safe and, if you're not a big fish eater, are probably a good idea because they contain lots of DHA (Docosahexanoic acid), good for your baby's eye and brain development.

WHERE TO GET YOUR OMEGA 3S

	g/100g	Portion	g/portion
Salmon	2.5g	100g	2.5g
Mackerel	2.8g	160g	4.5g
Sardines (tinned)	2.0g	100g	2.0g
Trout	1.3g	230g	2.9g
Tuna (canned in oil, drained)	1.1g	100g	1.1g
Cod liver oil	24g	1 teaspoon (5 ml)	1.2g
Flaxseed oil	57g	1 tablespoon (14g)	8.0g
Flaxseeds (ground)	16g	1 tablespoon (24g)	3.8g
Rapeseed oil	9.6g	1 tablespoon (14g)	1.3g
Walnuts	7.5g	1 tablespoon (28g)	2.6g
Walnut oil	11.5	1 tablespoon (14g)	1.6g
Pumpkin seeds	8.5g	2 tablespoons (25g)	2.1g
Omega 3 eggs		One egg	0.7g
Typical omega 3 supplement		8 capsules	0.5g

LOVE THE TRAILS?

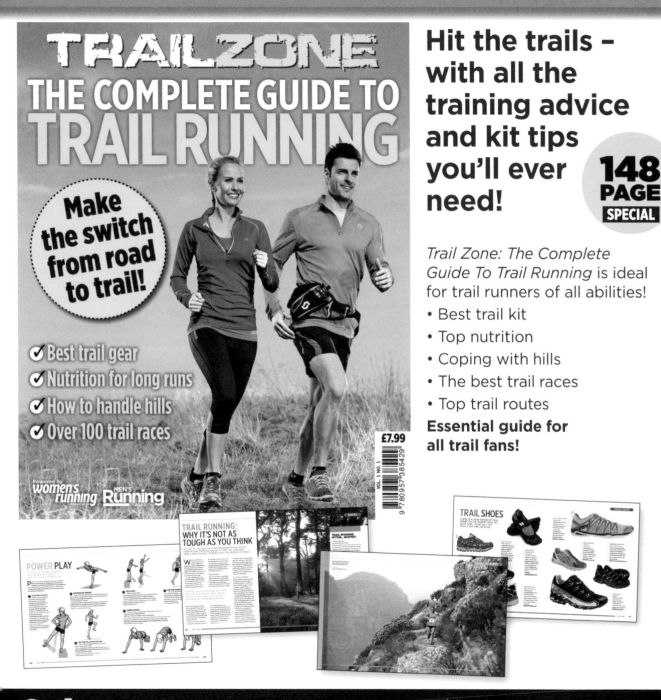

TRAILZONE

THE COMPLETE GUIDE TO TRAIL RUNNING

Make the switch from road to trail!

✓ Best trail gear
✓ Nutrition for long runs
✓ How to handle hills
✓ Over 100 trail races

Powered by
women's running magazine **MEN'S Running** magazine

£7.99

Hit the trails – with all the training advice and kit tips you'll ever need!

148 PAGE SPECIAL

Trail Zone: The Complete Guide To Trail Running is ideal for trail runners of all abilities!

• Best trail kit
• Top nutrition
• Coping with hills
• The best trail races
• Top trail routes

Essential guide for all trail fans!

IRON DEFICIENCY

IF YOU ARE FEMALE OR VEGETARIAN, OR SIMPLY NOT EATING ENOUGH OF THE RIGHT FOODS, YOU COULD BE IRON DEFICIENT. HERE'S HOW TO MAKE SURE YOU'RE GETTING ENOUGH

We all need iron. The recommended daily requirement is 14.8mg for women and only 8.7mg for men. (It's the only mineral that women need more of than men do.) In spite of this, surveys by the Food Standards Agency and the British Nutrition Foundation have consistently found that many British women don't get enough iron in their diet, resulting in the iron-deficiency symptoms of fatigue, poor concentration, pale complexion, brittle fingernails, headaches and poor appetite.

Iron is part of haemoglobin, the pigment that gives blood its red colour and which carries oxygen around the body in the blood. Active people, including runners, need a good supply of oxygen-rich blood to the muscles so it's especially important to be sure you're getting sufficient iron. However, there is quite a lot of evidence to show that female athletes, as well as other women who are especially active, may be short of iron.

WHY YOU MAY BE IRON DEFICIENT

There are several reasons why this happens. First of all, there's diet. As a nation, we are generally eating less and we're certainly eating less red meat – an excellent source of iron – than we were 40 years ago. Some nutritionists claim that the vegetables available today, even iron-rich ones, such as spinach, contain lower levels of vitamins and minerals than they did in the past. If you're on a restricted slimming or fad diet you may be at risk – the Food Standards Agency found that two in five teenage girls and a third of 19 to 24-year-olds had low iron stores. And if you're a vegetarian or a vegan, you need to plan your diet carefully if you are to obtain enough iron from your diet alone, and make sure you eat plenty of green vegetables, pulses and dried fruit. It is also important to remember that "haem iron", which is found in animal-derived products, is generally easier for the body to absorb than "non-haem iron" from vegetable sources.

It is not just how much iron-rich food you eat, it's also how well your body absorbs it. Some other foods can affect the absorption of iron, which is why nutritionists recommend you accompany your fortified breakfast cereal with a glass of orange juice rather than with a cup of tea. Vitamin C increases the absorption of iron, while the tannin in tea reduces it. If you want to maximise iron absorption, drink your tea or coffee at least half an hour after your meal. Some over-the-counter medicines, such as antacids, and also some prescription drugs, can affect iron absorption too.

Women may also run the risk of becoming iron-deficient if they have very heavy periods. "Heavy" means something different to every woman, but if you have to change your towel or tampon more often than every two hours, or if you regularly suffer from "flooding", a consultation with your GP or gynaecologist could be in order, to make sure you're not suffering from iron-deficiency anaemia.

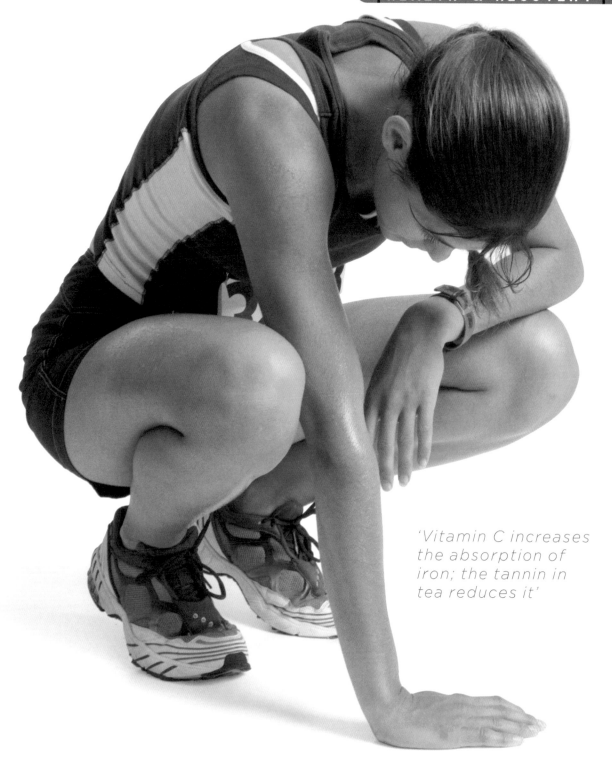

'Vitamin C increases the absorption of iron; the tannin in tea reduces it'

WHY DO RUNNERS BECOME IRON-DEFICIENT?

It seems that the pounding action of running can actually lead to the breakdown and eventual destruction of red blood cells, and therefore to loss of iron. High-impact exercise can sometimes result in trauma to the soles of the feet, known as "foot-strike haemolysis". You also lose a certain amount of iron when you perspire – it's been estimated that you lose 0.3-0.4mg of iron per litre of sweat during exercise! For all these reasons, it's important to ensure you have healthy haemoglobin levels.

HOW CAN YOU TELL IF YOUR IRON LEVELS ARE LOW?

The most common symptom is fatigue. If you just can't seem to drag yourself out of bed in the morning and your regular run begins to seem more like a chore than a pleasure, it could be that low iron stores are to blame. Looking pale, feeling faint and suffering from breathlessness can all be symptoms of iron deficiency, as can headaches, thinning hair and a tendency to catch every "bug" that's going round because of a depleted immune system.

If you suspect lack of iron might be causing your symptoms, ask your GP for a blood test, which will reveal whether or not you're short of iron. Don't take iron supplements unless your doctor prescribes them, because iron can be stored in the body and too much can be toxic, causing nausea, vomiting, stomach cramps and constipation.

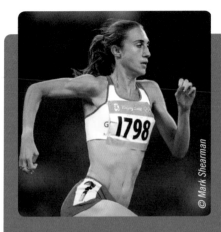

© Mark Shearman

'I felt drained and lethargic'

Lisa Dobriskey is one of the UK's best middle-distance runners. She took gold in the 2006 Commonwealth Games and silver in the 2009 world championships. She came fourth in the 1500m in the 2008 Beijing Olympics. But there was a time, not so long ago, when her training was not going at all as planned.

'I run about 70 miles a week when I'm training, as well as working with weights and on my general conditioning,' she says. 'The thought of going out on a cold morning is the worst part. Once I get my kit on and I'm out of the door it's not so bad. I'm usually up and running before the rest of the world gets going and I like that feeling. A couple of years ago, my training wasn't going well. I'd lost the urge to run, I felt drained and lethargic, and the more I did the worse I felt. My coach suggested I take a blood test and I found I had low iron levels. I was eating a balanced diet that had been recommended by a nutritionist, but endurance athletes often need supplements too, such as extra calcium and vitamin D.

'I began by taking iron supplements but they didn't agree with me. My local health food shop had SpaTone+, which is natural spring water already high in iron, so I tried that. It's very convenient to take – you can drink it as it is or add it to juice. Within a couple of weeks I was back on form, with plenty of energy. I started to look forward to my running again, just as I always had. Nothing was a chore or an effort – I felt great! I've learned a lot about how important iron is for female athletes. Those of us who are running up to 100 miles a week need to stay lean, and some people find it hard to absorb enough iron from their diets, especially if they don't eat much red meat.

'I don't worry too much about my diet – I just try to eat healthily, with plenty of fruit and vegetables, and fewer carbs in the summer. I'm not a big junk food eater, but I do love chocolate – a couple of squares is enough to satisfy my cravings!'

UP YOUR IRON INTAKE

Eat more:
- Lean red meat (it's the best source).
- Dark poultry meat, such as turkey and chicken legs.
- Eggs.
- Canned fish, such as tuna in oil, sardines and crab.
- Dried fruit, such as apricots and figs.
- Leafy green vegetables, including spinach, watercress, broccoli and savoy cabbage.
- Fortified breakfast cereals, such as bran flakes (check labels for information).

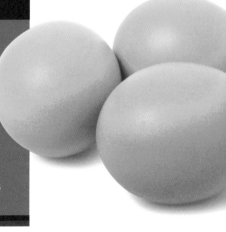

GET FIT FOR YOUR CHOSEN MARATHON WITH OUR GUIDE!

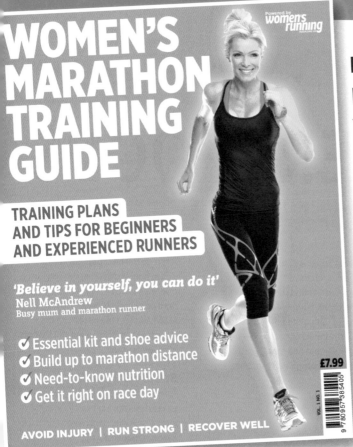

WOMEN'S MARATHON TRAINING GUIDE

Powered by women's running

TRAINING PLANS AND TIPS FOR BEGINNERS AND EXPERIENCED RUNNERS

'Believe in yourself, you can do it'
Nell McAndrew
Busy mum and marathon runner

- ✔ Essential kit and shoe advice
- ✔ Build up to marathon distance
- ✔ Need-to-know nutrition
- ✔ Get it right on race day

AVOID INJURY | RUN STRONG | RECOVER WELL

£7.99

EXPERT ADVICE!

Doing a marathon? Keep your training on track with top training advice, plans and nutritional tips from the experts at *Women's Running*. This **148-page** full-colour guide covers every aspect of marathon training, plus expert advice from model-turned-marathon runner Nell McAndrew.

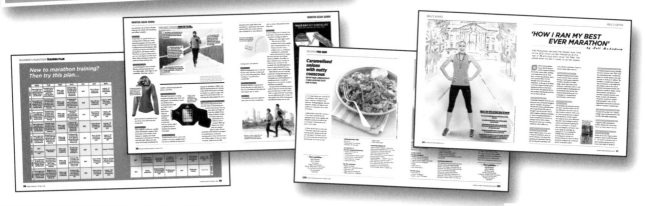

Order your copy now from only £7.24 online at www.amazon.co.uk

10 BEST RECOVERY FOODS

GET YOUR POST-RUN SNACK JUST RIGHT TO FEEL BETTER AND RECOVER FASTER

You've just finished a tough run and feel shattered, but before you put your feet up, you need to refuel those tired muscles. The quicker you consume food after a run, the quicker your body will recover. The ideal post-training snack should supply carbohydrate to replenish

'Raisins are a concentrated source of carbohydrate, which makes for a useful post-run snack when you need a quick energy boost. They are also a rich source of fibre, potassium and antioxidant vitamins and minerals'

depleted glycogen stores, as well as protein to repair and rebuild the muscles. Here are our top-ten foods for running recovery...

1: FLAVOURED MILK

Milk's high protein and carbohydrate content helps refuel exhausted muscles. A 2009 study from James Madison University in the US found that chocolate milk promoted better muscle recovery than a commercial

sports drink. And a 2008 study by researchers at Northumbria University found that athletes who drank 500ml of semi-skimmed milk or chocolate milk immediately after training suffered less muscle soreness and had more rapid muscle recovery compared with those who drank a commercial sports drink or plain water.
How much? 300-500ml.

2: YOGURT

Fruit yogurt contains carbohydrate (in the form of lactose and sucrose) and protein in a 4:1 ratio. According to University of Texas studies, this nutrient ratio accelerates post-exercise refuelling, which means faster recovery and muscles that feel

less sore the next day. Yogurt is also rich in bone-strengthening calcium – one 150g pot delivers around one third of your daily needs.
How much? One pot after runs lasting less than 30 minutes; two pots after longer runs.

3: CEREAL AND GRANOLA BARS

Cereal bars are easy to eat straight after a run when you haven't time for a meal. Choose bars containing lots of oats – for a more sustained energy boost – as well as a little more protein than other cereals. Most bars supply around 90 to 130 calories and less than 5g fat, which makes them quick to digest and a healthier option than biscuits.
How much? One bar following a 30-minute run; two bars after longer workouts.

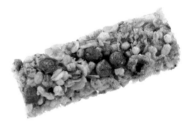

4: BANANAS

Bananas supply easily digestible carbohydrates – around 15g per banana – from a mixture of sugars (fructose, glucose and sucrose) and starch, which is perfect for replenishing muscle fuel. Bananas also deliver potassium, which is essential for balancing the fluid levels in your cells after running, and magnesium for making new body cells. Try blending one banana with a little honey and a cup of skimmed milk or a pot of yogurt for a nutritious smoothie.

How many? One banana for every 30 minutes of running.

5: RAISINS

Raisins are a concentrated source of carbohydrate, which makes for a useful post-run snack when you need a quick energy boost. They are also a rich source of fibre, potassium and antioxidant vitamins and minerals.

How much? A handful (60g) will speed up glycogen replenishment.

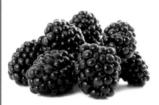

6: BLACKBERRIES

Avoid the risk of post-race colds by eating blackberries. Their high levels of natural phenolic acids help kill viruses and fight infections. About 15 berries provide one third of your daily requirements of vitamin C (for maintaining healthy cells) and half your vitamin E (helps relieve post-run soreness). Try this super quick dessert: whisk a 150ml pot of Greek or thick plain yogurt with a few drops of vanilla extract. Layer the yogurt with fresh blackberries and crunchy oat cereal in two sundae dishes.

How much? About 15 berries (or 85g) count as one of your five-a-day.

7: RICE CAKES WITH PEANUT BUTTER

Plain rice cakes can provide a quick energy boost after a run, but eating them with a little peanut butter is better. This combination provides the perfect ratio of carbs to protein (4:1) for speedy glycogen refuelling and muscle-protein repair. Peanut butter also provides protein, fibre and vitamin E.

How much? Four rice cakes with 20g (a tablespoon) of peanut butter.

8: NUTS

All nuts are a good source of protein, fibre, heart-protective vitamin E and B vitamins (which help release energy from food). They not only promote muscle recovery after a run, but they can also help you shed pounds. A study from Harvard Medical School found people who ate nuts as part of a Mediterranean-style diet lost more weight and kept it off longer than those who followed a traditional low-fat diet.

How much? Around 30g (a small handful) after running will aid muscle repair.

9: PANCAKES

Make your own or buy ready-made pancakes for a high-carb post-run snack. Two pancakes provide approximately 200 calories and 30g carbohydrate to refuel depleted muscles. They also supply 5-7g protein, which accelerates glycogen storage and rebuilds muscle cells. Top with a little honey or, for an added vitamin hit, a tablespoon of stewed apples.

How much? Two regular pancakes or four Scotch pancakes.

10: BAKED BEANS

Great for soluble fibre (the type that helps lower blood sugar and cholesterol levels), baked beans also give you 10g protein per average 200g serving, about the same as a large slice (40g) of cheese. Beans are also rich in iron, essential for transporting oxygen around the body, as well as B vitamins, zinc and magnesium. Eat them on toast, with a baked potato or, if you absolutely must, straight from the can!

How much? Half a tin (200g) gives you 27g carbs, the amount burned during a half-hour easy-pace run.

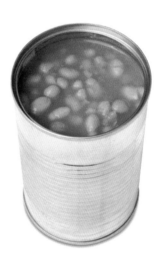

TOP 10 VITAMINS AND MINERALS FOR RUNNERS

YOU NEED MORE NUTRIENTS WHEN YOU'RE ACTIVE, BUT WHICH ARE THE MOST IMPORTANT AND HOW MUCH IS ENOUGH?

Regular intense exercise increases your requirements of the micronutrients involved in energy metabolism, tissue growth and repair, red blood cell manufacture and free radical defence. And while it's tempting to think supplements will boost your performance, there's little scientific evidence to support this theory. Most researchers conclude that a balanced diet should provide all the vitamins and minerals you need to train hard and stay healthy. Here's the low-down on the ten most useful.

1: VITAMIN E

Why you need it: Vitamin E is a powerful antioxidant that prevents the oxidation of fatty acids in cell membranes and protects your cells from the damage caused by strenuous exercise.

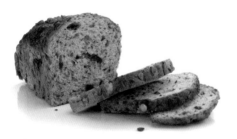

Best food sources: Vegetable oils, margarine, wholegrain bread, oily fish, nuts, seeds, avocado, green leafy vegetables and egg yolk.
How much? No Recommended Daily Allowance (RDA) in the UK, but the EU RDA is 10mg, which equals half an avocado, 80g spinach, six almonds or 10ml sunflower oil.

'Vitamin C is a potent antioxidant that can protect against exercise-related cell damage'

2: VITAMIN C

Why you need it: Vitamin C is needed for the growth and repair of body cells, and for the formation of connective tissues, red blood cells and exercise-related hormones, including adrenaline. It also promotes healthy blood vessels and strengthens the immune system. It's a potent antioxidant that can protect against exercise-related cell damage.

Best food sources? Fresh fruit and vegetables, particularly citrus fruit, berries and currants, and dark-green leafy vegetables.
How much? 40mg a day, which equals half an orange, half a red pepper or ten strawberries.

3: VITAMIN B6

Why you need it: This is involved in protein, fat and carbohydrate metabolism, which increases as a result of regular exercise. It's also needed for making red blood cells, new body proteins and antibodies.
Best food sources: Liver, nuts, pulses, eggs, bread, cereals, fish and bananas.
How much? 1.2mg: two bananas or 120g haddock.

4: FOLIC ACID

Why you need it: Folic acid is involved in the formation of red blood cells (runners have a higher red blood count than sedentary people) and is also needed for the manufacture of new body cells.
Best food sources: Dark-green leafy vegetables, oranges, fortified breakfast cereals and bread, yeast extract, nuts and pulses.
How much? 200 micrograms, which

equals 30g bran flakes, 25g peanuts or one serving (3g) of yeast extract.

5: VITAMIN A AND BETA-CAROTENE

Why you need it: Vitamin A helps you to see in dim light (important if you run in the dark); it promotes healthy skin, hair and eyes, and keeps the linings of organs, such as the lungs, in good condition. Beta-carotene, converted into vitamin A in the body, is an antioxidant that helps protect the cells from oxidative damage during intense exercise.

Best food sources:
Vitamin A – liver, cheese, oily fish, eggs, butter and margarine.
Beta-carotene – dark-green vegetables, and yellow, orange and red fruits.
How much? Vitamin A – 700 micrograms, which equals 15g margarine, one egg or two tablespoons of spinach. There's no RDA for beta-carotene.

6: CALCIUM

Why you need it: Calcium is important for the structure of bones and teeth, but it also plays an important role in blood clotting, muscle contraction and nerve function. Weight-bearing exercise, such as running, increases bone mass and calcium absorption, so it's important to get enough calcium in your diet.

Best food sources: Milk and dairy products, sardines, dark-green leafy vegetables, pulses, nuts and seeds.
How much? 700mg, which equals a glass (200ml) of milk, a pot (150g) of yogurt or two tinned sardines (40g).

7: IRON

Why you need it: Iron is important for runners as it's needed to make haemoglobin (which transports oxygen in the blood) and myoglobin (which transports oxygen in the muscle cells). A deficient intake can impair aerobic metabolism by decreasing delivery of oxygen to the muscles and reducing the ability of muscles to use oxygen for energy.

Best food sources: Meat and offal, wholegrain cereals, nuts, fortified breakfast cereals, beans, lentils and green leafy vegetables. Including vitamin C-rich foods with meals, for example, fruit with breakfast cereal, enhances absorption of iron.
How much? 14.8mg, which equals one steak (150g), 100g spinach, 100g salmon or a 45g bowl of bran flakes.

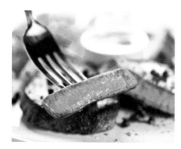

8: VITAMIN D

Why you need it: It's needed for strong bones (along with calcium and phosphorus), as it helps the body to absorb calcium.

Best food sources: Sunlight is actually the best source of vitamin D, but it's also found in oily fish, liver, eggs, fortified breakfast cereals and margarine.
How much? There's no RDA, but you should be able to get enough vitamin D by getting ten minutes of sun exposure a day on your face and arms. Pregnant and breastfeeding women need 10mcg.

9: ZINC

Why you need it: Zinc is crucial to the activity of more than 70 enzymes involved in the metabolism of proteins, fats and carbohydrates. It also helps heal wounds and promote recovery from soft-tissue injuries, as

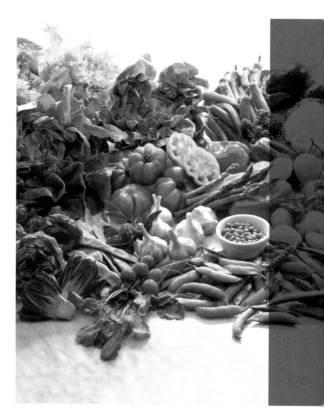

well as keeping the immune system healthy and fighting infection.
Best food sources: Nuts, lentils, beans, eggs, wholegrain cereals, meat, milk and dairy products.
How much? 7mg, which equals 115g steak, 85g cashew nuts, four slices of wholemeal bread or 115g cooked lentils.

10: MAGNESIUM

Why you need it: Magnesium is involved in tissue repair, and muscle and nerve function. It also helps the body absorb calcium and potassium, and utilise vitamins B6, C and E.
Best food sources: Wholegrain cereals, nuts, fruit, vegetables and dark chocolate.
How much? 270mg (women) or 300mg (men), which equals 50g mixed nuts, three slices of wholemeal bread, two shredded wheat or 50g dark chocolate.

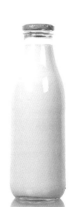

VEGGIE MIGHT

IF YOU DON'T EAT MEAT, MAKE SURE YOU DON'T MISS OUT ON THE VITAL NUTRIENTS THAT WILL BOOST YOUR RUNNING

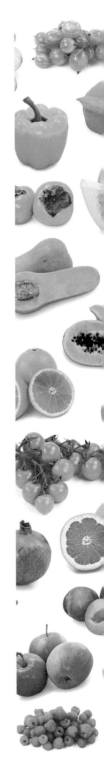

Whether you choose to go vegetarian for the health benefits, for environmental reasons or out of moral conviction, getting the nutrients your body needs can be challenging, especially if you run on a regular basis. Here's how to avoid the dietary pitfalls.

WHAT MAKES A VEGETARIAN?

The term vegetarian is used more broadly than its true definition. A vegetarian diet excludes meat, poultry and fish. A lacto-ovo vegetarian diet includes dairy products and eggs, while a vegan doesn't eat dairy products or eggs. The terms "demi-vegetarian" or "pescatarian" are sometimes used to mean diets that exclude red meat but include fish (in the case of pescatarians), poultry, dairy products and eggs.

HOW WILL A VEGETARIAN DIET AFFECT MY RUNNING PERFORMANCE?

Many studies report that vegetarian diets can support sports performance. A 2009 review by the American Dietetic Association concluded the nutritional needs of athletes can be met by well-planned vegetarian diets. It's not clear whether a vegetarian diet will improve athletic performance, however, as there haven't been any studies to date that have controlled the inherent differences between vegetarian and non-vegetarian diets. A 2006 US study did point out that vegetarian athletes generally have higher levels of vitamin C, vitamin E and beta-carotene than non-vegetarians, which may help reduce exercise-related stress on the body. Reassuringly, other studies have shown that excluding meat from your diet will not impair aerobic fitness or endurance performance.

AVOID THE PITFALLS

As a non-meat eater, you need to make up for the nutrients you'd otherwise get from meat. If you don't include suitable vegetarian alternatives, you risk insufficient intakes of certain nutrients crucial for health and performance. Although a vegetarian diet can provide all the essential nutrients to support intense daily training, there are several dietary challenges you face.

IF YOU'RE VEGAN...
Calories

A vegan diet is usually higher in fibre and more bulky than a diet that contains meat and dairy, which means it may not contain enough calories to support hard training. If you need 3,000 calories a day, you'll need to eat plenty of energy-dense foods, such as nuts, peanut butter, seeds, tofu, soya and Quorn.

Protein

If you omit meat, dairy and eggs, you need to substitute a plant protein: beans, lentils, nuts, seeds, soya products, cereals and Quorn. Single plant foods do not contain all the essential amino acids you need in the right proportions, so they should be combined to ensure all amino acids are consumed. You don't need to include complementary proteins at each meal, as long as you eat a good variety of protein sources throughout the day.

Vitamin B12

This is needed for making red blood cells and to maintain the covering around nerve fibres, but is found exclusively in animal products. If you're vegan, you need to eat B12-fortified foods, such as soya milk, breakfast cereals and yeast extract, or fermented soya foods, such as miso and tempeh, or take a supplement.

Calcium

If you don't consume dairy, it's more difficult to get your calcium quota. Aim to include at least three daily servings of dark-green vegetables (such as spinach or curly kale), calcium-enriched soya milk or cheese, nuts, seeds, tofu or dried figs.

IF YOU'RE VEGETARIAN...
Iron

While green leafy vegetables, wholegrains and beans all contain some iron, the body doesn't absorb it as well as it does iron from animal sources. Including vitamin C-rich foods (fruit and fresh green vegetables) with your meals will increase iron absorption. However, phytates and oxalates in bran cereals and spinach can block iron getting

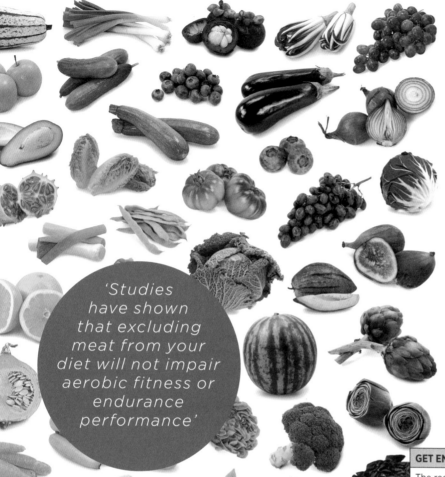

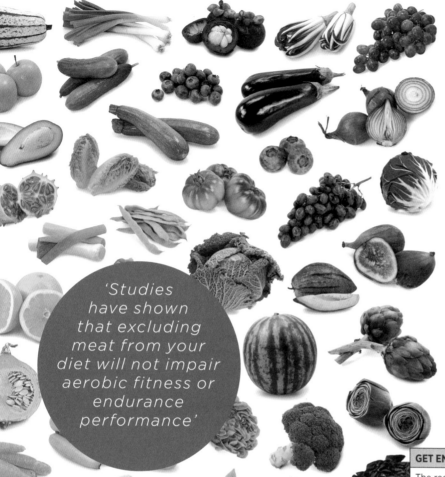

> 'Studies have shown that excluding meat from your diet will not impair aerobic fitness or endurance performance'

into your bloodstream, as can tannin in tea. Aim to get at least two daily servings of lentils, beans, nuts, curly kale, dried fruit and fortified breakfast cereals.

Zinc

To get enough zinc, eat three daily servings of wholegrains (although large quantities of wholegrains can actually reduce zinc absorption), seeds, beans, lentils and dark green leafy vegetables. Dairy products, peas and potatoes also contain zinc.

Omega 3 fats

If you don't eat fish, you'll need to get your omega 3s from plant foods rich in the fatty acid ALA: nuts, seeds and dark-green leafy veg, such as kale and spinach. The omega 3 oils in these foods are less potent than those in fish, but are still valuable to the body. The Vegetarian Society recommends consuming 4g of ALA a day, equivalent to 50g walnuts, 2tsp flaxseed oil or 2½ tbsp rapeseed oil.

EAT SUFFICIENT CALCIUM

The recommended daily allowance for calcium is 700mg. Use the following table to make sure your intake is sufficient.

FOOD	700MG CALCIUM
Milk	1 glass (170ml)
Cheddar cheese	1 slice (25g)
Yogurt	1 carton (130g)
Broccoli	10 stalks (500g)
Oranges	3 oranges
Almonds	50 nuts (83g)
Dried figs	4 figs (80g)
Tofu	1 slice (40g)

GET ENOUGH IRON

The recommended daily allowance for iron is 14.8mg. Use the following table to make sure your intake is sufficient.

FOOD	IRON CONTENT (MILLIGRAMS/ PORTION)
140g steak	2.9
130g chicken breast	0.8
100g canned sardines	2.3
3 tbsp (120g) cooked red lentils	2.9
200g baked beans	2.8
2 eggs	1.6
2 slices wholemeal bread	1.3
100g broccoli	1.0
100g spinach	1.7

THE GOOD FAT GUIDE

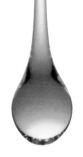

NOT ALL FATS ARE BAD. MAKE THE RIGHT CHOICES AND YOU COULD BOOST YOUR RUNNING PERFORMANCE

Do you avoid fat because you think it will hinder your running or make you gain weight? In fact, eating too little of certain types of fat may hinder your performance, increase your risk of health problems or injury and suppress your immune system. If less than 20 per cent of your total calorie intake comes from fat you may be missing out on the good fats found in vegetable oils, seeds, nuts and oily fish. These fats assist vitamin absorption, lower blood cholesterol, control blood pressure and help regulate your metabolism.

HOW MUCH FAT SHOULD YOU EAT?

The amount of fat recommended for good health for the general UK population is 15 to 35 per cent of energy, or a maximum of 70g a day if you consume 2,000 calories; 95g a day if you consume 2,500 calories. Higher intakes may increase your risk

of developing obesity, high blood cholesterol levels, heart disease and stroke.

But for runners, there's no specific guidance. The International Olympic Committee and International Association of Athletic Federations both recommend athletes focus their efforts on getting enough carbohydrate and protein. The balance of your calorie intake should come from fats – ideally "good" rather than "bad" fats. These will provide numerous health benefits as well as a source of energy.

WHAT ARE GOOD AND BAD FATS?

"Good" fats are the unsaturated fats – monounsaturates and polyunsaturates, found in fish, nuts, seeds and olives (and their oils). "Bad" fats are saturated fats and trans fats, which have been linked to increased risk of heart disease and cancer.

'Omega 3 enhances oxygen delivery to working muscles, boosts your endurance and prevents injury'

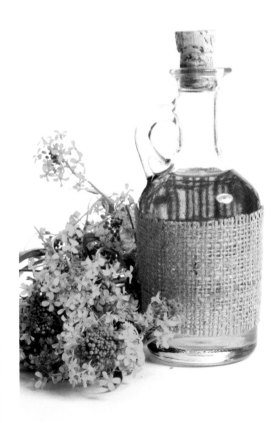

GOOD FATS	BAD FATS
Monounsaturated fats: olive oil, rapeseed oil, avocados, nuts, peanut butter	Saturated fats: fatty meats, burgers, sausages, butter, palm oil, biscuits, cakes, cheese
Polyunsaturated fats: sunflower oil, corn oil, sunflower margarine, nuts, seeds	Trans fats: some margarines and spreads, biscuits, pastries, pies, cakes, takeaway fried food
Omega 3 fats: sardines, salmon, mackerel, pilchards, walnuts, pumpkin seeds, eggs	

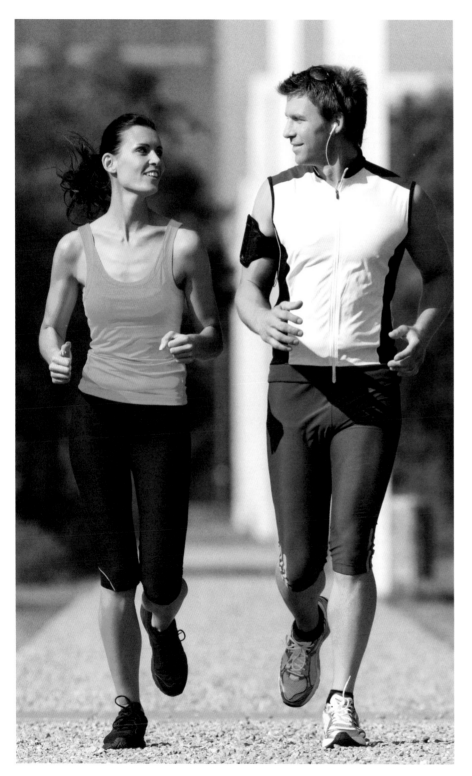

THE GOOD GUYS

Monounsaturated fats help lower "bad" LDL cholesterol levels while maintaining levels of "good" HDL, which helps cut heart disease and cancer risk. They are found in olive oil, rapeseed and soya oil, avocados, nuts, peanut butter, and seeds.

Polyunsaturated fats include omega 3 and omega 6 fats. Omega 3 fatty acids are alpha linolenic acid (ALA, found in walnuts, pumpkin seeds, flax seeds and rapeseed oil), eicosapentaenoic acid (EPA) and docosahexaenoic acid (DHA), the latter two both found only in oily fish (sardines, mackerel, salmon, fresh tuna, trout, herring). In the body, ALA can be converted into EPA and DHA, which are needed for the proper functioning of the brain; protect against heart disease and stroke; and may help prevent memory loss and treat depression. The minimum requirement is 0.9g a day, which you can get from one portion (140g) of oily fish a week or one tablespoon of omega 3-rich oil daily.

Omega 6 fatty acids – linoleic acid and gamma linolenic acid (GLA) – are found in sunflower, safflower, corn, groundnut and olive oils, and margarine-type spreads made with them; peanuts and peanut butter, sunflower and sesame seeds. Most people get plenty of omega 6s but not enough omega 3s.

THE BAD GUYS

Saturated fats are found in animal fats as well as products made with palm oil. They have no beneficial role in the body (apart from being a source of energy); they raise blood cholesterol and increase the risk of heart disease. However, it would be impractical to cut them out altogether, so stick to an intake less than the guideline daily amount (GDA): 30g for men and 20g for women. Sources include fatty meats, full-fat dairy products, butter, lard, palm oil and palm kernel oil (both labelled as "vegetable fat" on foods); biscuits, cakes and desserts made with palm or palm kernel oil or vegetable fat.

Trans fats are formed during the commercial process of hydrogenation, which converts unsaturated oils into solid spreads (hydrogenated fats or oils) for making biscuits, desserts and pastry. Trans fats increase LDL ("bad") cholesterol levels and lower HDL ("good") cholesterol, harden and stiffen the arteries which increases the heart disease risk.

Try to avoid these fats completely by checking for hydrogenated oils and partially hydrogenated oils on the ingredients list on food packages.

GOOD FATS FOR BETTER RUNNING

One group of fats, the omega 3 fatty acids, are especially good for runners, enhancing oxygen delivery to working muscles, boosting your endurance and preventing ligament, joint and tendon strains.

Studies show that omega 3s increase blood flow and the delivery of oxygen to muscles, which can lead to faster improvements in aerobic fitness. Regular exercisers who supplemented their diet with fish

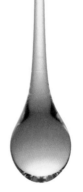

oil supplements (4g omega 3s per day) for ten weeks increased their maximal oxygen consumption (VO2 max) by 11 per cent, compared with controls who did not take supplements, in a study carried out at Western Washington University.

Oxygen delivery to active muscles and enhanced blood flow can be factors that delay fatigue during activity. A 2004 study of runners found a correlation between omega 3 intake and increased exercise time before fatigue.

Good fats can also help reduce inflammation and muscle soreness following a hard run, speed recovery and reduce joint stiffness. A 2009 study found that people who took fish oil for 30 days had significantly less post-exercise muscle soreness and inflammation after a single 40-minute exercise session compared with those who took a placebo.

Other studies have found that omega 3s can improve lung function in people who suffer from exercise-induced asthma.

OTHER BENEFITS OF OMEGA 3 FATS

Large-scale studies have suggested that a higher intake of omega 3s and fish are linked to a lower risk of heart disease and stroke, a reduced risk of bowel and breast cancer and

increased immune function. They may also help symptoms of rheumatoid arthritis, asthma, eczema and inflammatory bowel disease, all conditions that are associated with an exaggerated inflammatory response and unbalanced immune function. While running can boost your mood and promote psychological wellbeing (by boosting levels of endorphins), omega 3s may further enhance these benefits. Supplementation with omega 3s has been shown to reduce symptoms of depression. People with higher levels of omega 3s in the blood are more likely to maintain cognitive function as they age and have a lower risk of dementia.

CHANGE YOUR WAYS

▸▸ Focus on good fats (monounsaturated, polyunsaturated and omega 3 fats) and minimise the ones that can harm your health (saturated and trans fats).
▸▸ Aim to consume around 0.5 to 1g good fats per kilogram of bodyweight.
▸▸ Choose olive or rapeseed oil for cooking, use sesame, flaxseed or walnut oil for dressings, smear hummus or peanut butter instead of butter on your bread, and add one of the following to your daily menu: half an avocado, two tablespoons of nuts or seeds, a portion of sardines or salmon, or a tablespoon of olive oil.

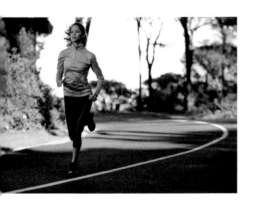

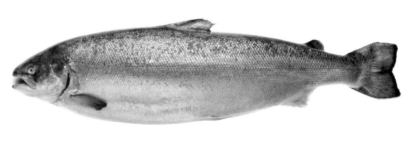

REGISTER TODAY FOR THE
WOMEN'S RUNNING E-NEWSLETTER

With our features, forums and exclusive competitions, the *Women's Running* online community is the place for you!

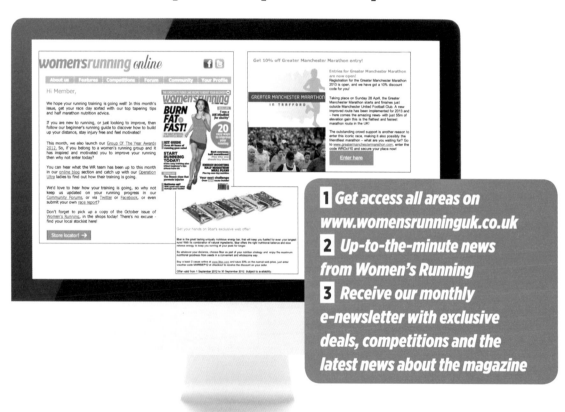

1 *Get access all areas on www.womensrunninguk.co.uk*

2 *Up-to-the-minute news from Women's Running*

3 *Receive our monthly e-newsletter with exclusive deals, competitions and the latest news about the magazine*

Register today!

To enjoy all the best features of the website, follow our fast, simple registration process. You'll be able to access new areas of the site and can receive our free newsletter too

www.womensrunninguk.co.uk

OUR PROMISE – we will never sell or rent your details to third parties

EAT TO PROTECT YOUR JOINTS

SUPPORT YOUR JOINTS AND MINIMISE INFLAMMATION WITH THESE SIX SUPER-PROTECTORS

Running doesn't need to spell an end to healthy joints. In fact, regular running strengthens the muscles surrounding your joints, tendons and ligaments, helping to prevent injuries.

But to further protect your joints, you need to avoid overtraining and schedule adequate recovery time into your training plan. You also need to have a balanced diet that incorporates enough carbohydrate and protein to fuel your training and assist with muscle repair. There are also a few extra-special ingredients that have been shown to support the body's healing process and reduce inflammation. So, if you'd rather be out and about on regular runs than nursing an injury, read on for our list of super-protectors – the nutritional marvels that will help support your joints and keep you on the road.

WATER
Staying hydrated during and after exercise helps to minimise inflammation in the body, which will improve your ability to recover from your training sessions. Dehydration places extra stress on the immune system, as well as increasing your likelihood of developing tendon and ligament injuries, so make sure you drink up after your run. You should aim to replace approximately 800ml of water for each hour of exercise, adding electrolytes (the salts you lose in sweat) to your drink if you've been running for 90 minutes or more.

OMEGA 3
Omega 3 essential fatty acids, found in oily fish, walnuts, flax seeds and pumpkin seeds, are great for keeping inflammation at bay. The National Institute of Health recommends that approximately two per cent of your total daily calories come from omega 3 fats. To meet these recommendations, a person consuming 2,000 calories a day should eat enough omega 3-rich foods to take in 4g of omega 3 each day (if you're pregnant or planning to have a baby, don't eat more than two portions of oily fish each week). If you're not getting enough from your diet, take a good-quality omega 3 supplement.

FRESH FRUIT AND VEGETABLES
We all know fruit and vegetables are good for us, supplying plenty of vitamins and minerals. But brightly coloured fruits and vegetables also provide antioxidants and flavanols, known for their anti-inflammatory properties, so try to include them in most of your meals.

BROMELAIN
Found in pineapples, bromelain, a mixture of enzymes, has an anti-inflammatory effect (it has been in use for centuries as medicine in Central and South America). If you're putting in the miles or have increased the

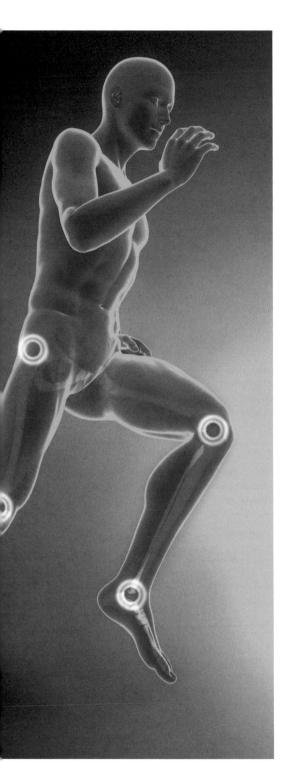

intensity of your training, you may benefit from snacking on pineapple between meals.

QUERCETIN

This active ingredient, found in apples and red onions, has also been shown to reduce inflammation. So, it's worth sticking to the old adage "an apple a day", or simply add red onions to casseroles or sauces.

GLUCOSAMINE

When you damage tissue, your body reacts by producing glucosamine (which naturally occurs in tendons, ligaments and cartilage) to form new connective molecules. Glucosamine's main function is to stimulate the growth of cartilage and hydrate tendons and ligaments, protecting them from injury. The body normally manufactures this miracle hydrator and protector, but as production levels diminish with age or because of excessive training, glucosamine levels can fall short of what you need, leaving your joints, tendons and ligaments vulnerable.

Taking a glucosamine supplement will increase the synthesis of a substance called chondroitin, which keeps your cartilage nourished, hydrated and strong. When looking for a glucosamine joint formula, select a product that combines glucosamine and chondroitin, which will restore synovial fluid and tissues in and around your joints, cushioning the bones, tendons and ligaments from damage. The ideal dose is 520mg of glucosamine and 300mg of chondroitin per day – they can be found in all good health food shops.

If you want to avoid injury, improving your diet and including these foods can form part of your protective programme. Investing in

'Brightly coloured fruit and vegetables provide antioxidants and flavanols, known for their anti-inflammatory properties, so try to include them in most meals'

regular massage and physiotherapy can help, too, as will adding core-stability work and stretching to your training programme. Making time for these lifestyle changes, as well as factoring adequate rest into your programme and avoiding pushing yourself too far, too soon, will make sure you enjoy injury-free running all year round.

GUT REACTION

WE'VE ALL HEARD OF RUNNER'S TROTS, BUT JUST HOW DO YOU STOP THEM INTERFERING WITH YOUR TRAINING? HERE ARE THE BEST WAYS TO ALLEVIATE TUMMY TROUBLES

It's not the most wholesome of topics, we know. But our collective coyness cannot disguise the fact that digestive issues affect a huge proportion of runners.

Exercise is hugely beneficial for our insides – research shows daily activity can alleviate constipation and, long-term, reduce your risk of colon cancer by around 24 per cent. But there is a flip side – studies suggest up to half of all athletes regularly

'Up to half of all athletes regularly experience varying degrees of intestinal upset'

experience varying degrees of intestinal upset, from nausea and flatulence to cramping and diarrhoea. And, sadly, runners are particularly vulnerable – frequency of digestive issues is almost twice that of cyclists or swimmers.

This seems to be caused by a combination of factors. 'When we run, blood is diverted away from the intestines to the legs and we move in an up-and-down motion,' says Dr David Sanders, medical advisor for digestive disorders charity Core (www.corecharity.org.uk). 'Together, the two factors – particularly the bouncing movement of running – seem to have a stimulating impact.' And the more pronounced the motion of the body (for instance, during speed or interval training), the worse it can be. It's not just uncomfortable and embarrassing – it can affect your performance, too. You don't need us to tell you that abdominal cramps and loo stops put the brakes on progress.

BOLSTER YOUR BOWELS

You can't always control your bowels, but you can watch what you're putting in them. Follow some common-sense dietary advice to rein in your wayward digestion. Try to avoid eating for at least two hours before you exercise and bypass anything that's hard for your body to digest. 'By default, energy-rich meals can also be high in fibre,' says Dr Sanders. 'For those who suffer with "runner's trots", it's best to avoid fibrous pre-run meals, such as bran-based breakfast cereals.' Stick to easy-on-your-gut snacks, such as plain bagels, and low-fibre fresh fruit and veg, such as melon, lettuce and tomatoes.

Spicy and fatty foods, acidic fruit such as pineapple, alcohol and fizzy drinks cause gut woes even in couch potatoes, so definitely give them a wide berth before a run. 'Keep a food diary and identify your particular digestive triggers,' adds Dr Sanders. On a practical level, try to time your workouts according to your usual bowel movements and factor in possible toilet stops when planning your routes – use www.findatoilet. co.uk to find public conveniences along the way. And don't forget to take water with you to rehydrate should a bout of diarrhoea strike.

RACE STRATEGY
Don't let your bowels ruin your big day!
➤ As part of your training, devote some time to testing different meals and energy drinks or gels (the sweeteners can play havoc), so you don't have a nasty shock on race day. Check on the race website about the toilet facilities along the route.

NATURAL BOWEL CALMERS

SOOTHE YOUR PRE- AND POST-RUN DIGESTION THE ALTERNATIVE WAY

PEPPERMINT: Studies show that peppermint oil helps up to a half of IBS sufferers, relieving wind and preventing painful spasms. Try Holland & Barrett Enteric Coated Oil of Peppermint Capsules, £6.49 for 90. (www.hollandandbarrett.com).

GINGER: It's an age-old digestive aid and a recent study also found ginger can ease muscle pain. Try it candied, ground or in tea. We like Pukka's Three Ginger Tea, £2.29 for 20 sachets (www.pukkaherbs.com).

Aloe Vera juice: Refreshing, tangy and ultra-calming, Aloe Vera juice can be added as a shot to your juices and smoothies. Try Holland & Barrett's Aloe Vera Juice, £11.55 for 946ml.

PROBIOTICS: The good intestinal flora in probiotics can help prevent diarrhoea or reinvigorate your insides if you've already suffered. Try as a drink – Symprove, £21.95 for one bottle (www.symprove.com); or as a capsule – Viridian High Strength Tri-Blend Acidophilus Complex, £28.50 for 30 capsules (www.viridian-nutrition.com).

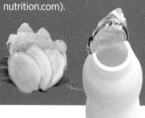

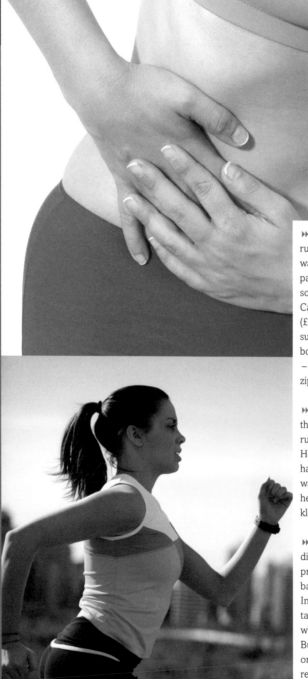

▸▸ Get yourself a lightweight running pouch to sling around your waist and pack a few sheets of loo paper and a compact sanitising gel, so your hands stay germ-free. Try Carex Hand Gel Sensitive 50ml (£1.45, available nationwide). Make sure the kit you're wearing on your bottom half is easy to remove – the last thing you need is a fiddly zip or buckle!

▸▸ Warm caffeinated drinks can get things moving downstairs, so some runners favour a pre-race espresso. However, don't over-indulge if you have a sensitive stomach. And sip water prudently, otherwise you'll be heading for the loo as soon as the klaxon sounds.

▸▸ 'If you know you're prone to diarrhoea, consider packing a product like Imodium in your race bag,' recommends Dr Sanders. Try Imodium Instants (£3.45 for six tablets, available nationwide), which are easy to take on the move. But don't become overly dependent on medication – use it only as a last resort. With time, patience and lifestyle changes, you can train your bowels to be more obedient.

RUNNING &
WEIGHT LOSS

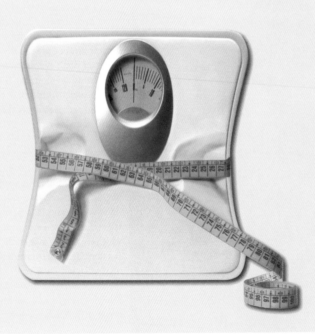

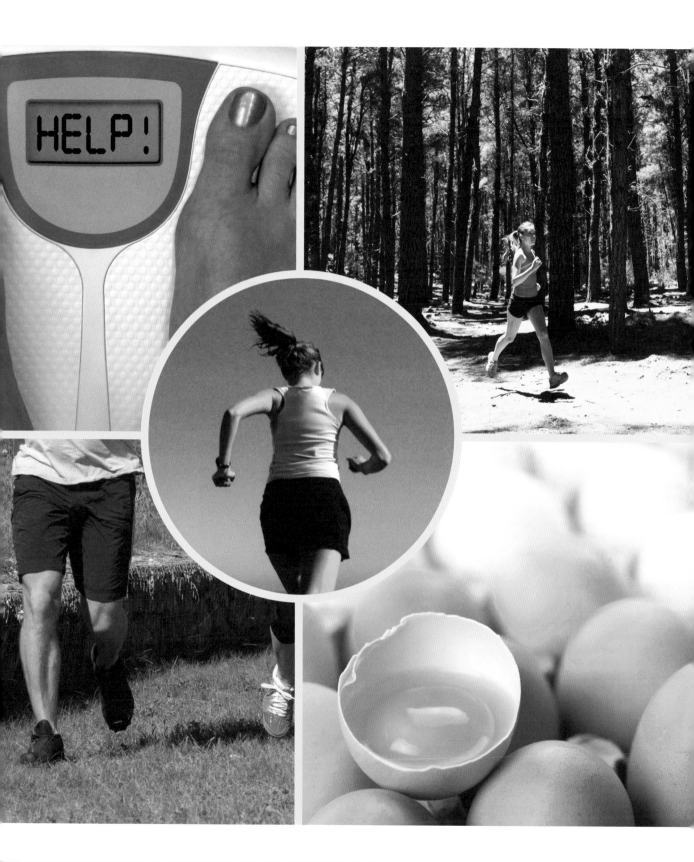

FILL UP NOT OUT!

CAN'T SEEM TO SATISFY THOSE HUNGER PANGS? TUCK INTO FOODS WITH A HIGH SATIETY VALUE AND FEEL FULLER FOR LONGER

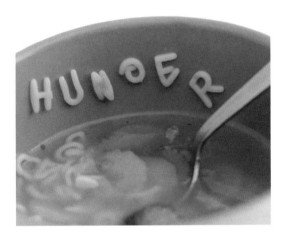

When you're trying to lose a few pounds, it's those pesky but all too familiar hunger pangs that are the most common reason for throwing in the towel and scoffing a pack of chocolate chip cookies. Yet by choosing your foods more carefully and including plenty of those that fill you up but not out, you can stay fuller for longer and curb the cravings that lead to calorie overload. Interestingly, scientists have found you tend to eat about the same amount of food every day, with how full you feel being based on the weight and/or volume of food you eat, not its calorie content.

One of the key ways to feel full and stay trim is to build your diet around low energy-density foods – those that provide plenty of weight and bulk, but with few calories. Choosing foods that are higher in protein, fibre and complex carbohydrates can also

trigger satiety mechanisms and help curb hunger more effectively. To feel optimally full on fewer calories, here's our list of top ten filling foods...

BOILED POTATOES

In the now world-famous satiety index created back in the nineties at the University of Sydney, boiled potatoes were top of the fullness scale, ranking three times more satisfying than white bread. Not all potatoes are created equal, though: chips, with their higher fat content, score much lower in their ability to satisfy.

EGGS

Eating two high-protein scrambled eggs for breakfast contributed to greater satiety compared with bagel consumption up to the same calorie level, according to a study from America's Louisiana State University.

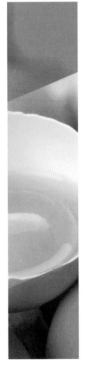

What's more, participants' energy intake was reduced over the following 36 hours, and blood cholesterol levels remained unchanged.

FISH

Fish is high in protein, which, gram for gram, is a better appetite buster than carbohydrate or fat. Moreover, fish, especially white fish, such as cod, haddock or pollock, has fewer calories than meat, which means you can eat a bigger portion. Try jazzing up grilled or poached white fish with a chunky tomato sauce laced with a little chilli.

PORRIDGE

Porridge proved to be twice as satisfying as Special K on the University of Sydney's satiety index. Instant porridge only needs a boiled kettle to be ready in no time at all, and is great if you're on the run. If you

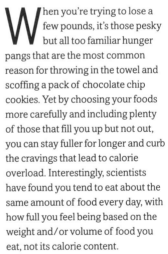

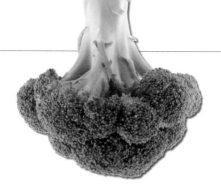

have a little more time, add interest with cinnamon, a drizzle of honey or your favourite dried fruit. You can even cook porridge in a slow cooker overnight, so you wake up to a hearty start to the day.

BROCCOLI

Of course all green veg is healthy and low calorie, but broccoli stands out in the stomach-filling stakes because it's bulkier than other veg, taking up room on your plate and in your stomach. Compare a Mars bar with ten large portions of broccoli – they both contain around 280 calories – and you can see how the broccoli will fill you up far more. And it's a fabulous source of vitamins and antioxidants, too.

CHICKEN NOODLE SOUP

Listed by the British Nutrition Foundation (www.nutrition.org.uk) as one of the lower energy-density foods, chicken noodle soup (or you could choose minestrone or any other non-creamy soup) is the ultimate filling-but-not-fattening food. Satiety expert Dr Barbara Rolls of Pennsylvania State University found people consumed an average 100 fewer calories when offered chicken and rice in a soup rather than as a casserole, or as a chicken and rice dish with a separate glass of water.

AIR-POPPED POPCORN

Popcorn has stomach-filling volume and, provided you avoid buttered, toffee or sugared types, it can fill you wonderfully well without ruining your diet. You'll be surprised how delicious air popped corn can be, especially when it's still warm. For calorie-free sweetness, try sprinkling over some granular artificial sweetener, or try curry powder for a savoury treat.

APPLES

All fruits are wonderfully filling foods, but apples are particularly convenient and portable, and the pectin fibre they contain swells in the digestive system, giving them the edge as a low-calorie satiating food. If you're tempted by a biscuit, have one of these versatile fruits instead.

WHOLE WHEAT SPAGHETTI

Plain, unfilled pasta is a filling food, whole wheat varieties particularly so. The low-glycaemic index (GI) will keep hunger curbed for a decent time, but do keep an eye on portion size – pasta is satisfying, precisely because you don't need to eat lots of it to feel full. A fist-sized portion is about right.

CANNED BEANS

All pulses have a very low GI, meaning they release their energy slowly and are among the best appetite-curbing foods in existence. You can pop them in soups and casseroles for extra bulk without adding many calories. Good old baked beans count, too.

'One of the key ways to feel full and stay trim is to eat low energy-density foods – those that provide plenty of weight and bulk, but few calories'

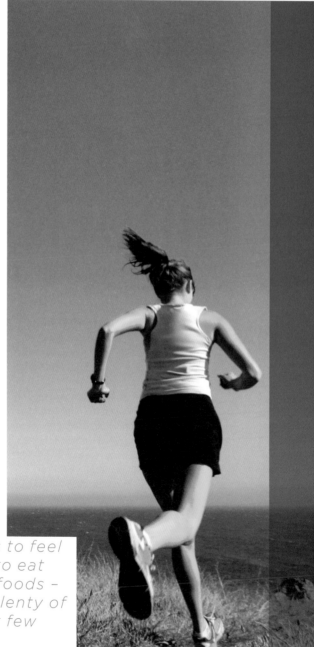

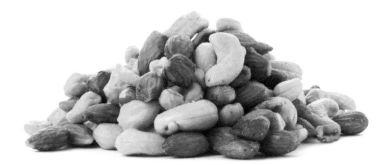

FOODS WITH HIDDEN CALORIES

EVEN HEALTHY FOOD CAN LEAD TO WEIGHT GAIN IF YOU'RE NOT CAREFUL

Low fat! All natural! One of your five a day! No added sugar! Sugar free! We've heard it all before. Most of what we know about the nutritional value of food comes from what we see on television or read on food packaging. But don't be under any illusions: manufacturers want you to buy their products and if they think sales can be increased if they brand something as healthy, however dubious the claim, they will do so.

'Despite all the campaigns to make breakfast cereals healthy, they still contain a lot of calories'

Recently, a group of nutritionists warned that basic calorie labelling is misleading, meaning that many people are eating more calories than they think. 'There is a lot of misinformation around calories, and it is crucial for the consumer, whether they are on a diet or not, to have the correct information about what they eat,' says Professor Richard Wrangham of Harvard University. He says the public is being given 'erroneous information about the energy value of many foods'.

And that's presuming people read the detailed nutrition information, which most of us do not have the time to do. Then there are the issues of food additives, portion sizes, hidden sugars and basic, natural assumptions (fruit's good, right? Yes, but it's not that simple…) and you end up with a

food minefield. Let us take you safely through it…

TEN HEALTHY FOODS THAT CAN CAUSE WEIGHT GAIN

OLIVE OIL

Olive oil can help reduce bad cholesterol and improve your immune system, but pouring it over every salad and adding it to every dish is a bad idea, as each tablespoon contains 119 calories. So just four tablespoons of olive oil adds up to almost a quarter of a women's recommended daily calorie consumption. Go easy.

FRUIT JUICES

Would you eat three oranges in one go? Probably not, but a 250ml glass

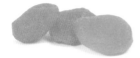

of 100 per cent orange juice, made from the juice of those three oranges, contains around 110 calories.

DRIED FRUIT

When you take the fluid out of food to produce dried fruit, you increase its calorie content. Avoid eating heaps of dried fruit, as it is very easy to consume half of your recommended daily amount of calories in just one snack.

NUTS

They're healthy – a great source of protein and plant oils – but they are very calorific. Limit yourself to one or two tablespoons at one go, to ensure you stay within your daily allowance.

SPREADS

Nutella and peanut butter are marketed as healthy and although they contain high levels of protein, they also contain more calories than jam. One teaspoon (10g) of peanut butter contains 62 calories.

BANANAS

Bananas pack a huge nutritional punch, but one medium banana contains 100 calories. To burn those off you'd need to run for about ten minutes.

YOGURTS

You might be surprised to see yogurt on the list, but with the large variety available on supermarket shelves you need to take care when choosing one. A small pot of yogurt can contain up to 250 calories.

BREAKFAST CEREALS

Despite all the campaigns to make breakfast cereals healthy, they still contain a lot of calories. The recommended portion size is 30g, which contains 110 calories. By increasing your portion size to 50g,

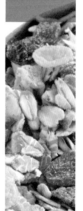

you increase your calorie intake by 75 calories per portion.

SMOOTHIES

As with juices, it's very easy to increase your calorie intake with smoothies. By combining milk, fruit, vegetables and protein powders in your favourite blend, you can easily hit 400 calories. If you use a smoothie as a meal replacement you will be fine, but as a snack the calorie content will be too high.

SALAD DRESSINGS

Some salad dressings can increase the calories of a healthy meal to more than that contained in a hamburger with chips. Three teaspoons of salad dressing contains 50 to 85 calories and there are more than three teaspoons in the pots of salad dressing that come with supermarket salads. Be careful when you choose your dressing and use it sparingly.

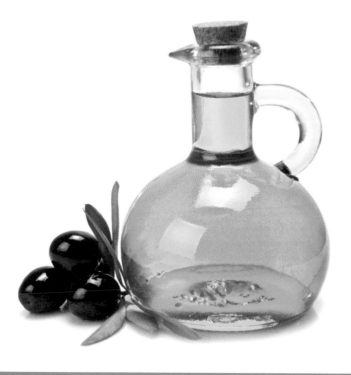

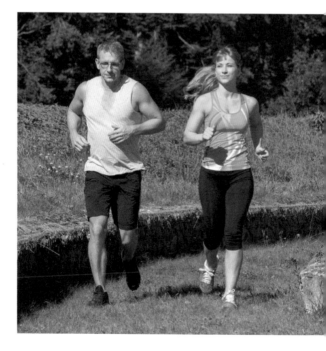

ARE YOU AT RISK OF DEVELOPING AN EATING DISORDER?

MANY PEOPLE RUN TO LOSE WEIGHT – BUT HOW DO YOU KNOW IF YOU'VE GONE TOO FAR? WE EXPLORE THE LINK BETWEEN RUNNING AND DISORDERED EATING

Attaining a healthy weight can lead to an improvement in running performance. But as the weight falls off, it can be easy to become obsessed with losing pounds. Many studies show runners have higher-than-average body dissatisfaction and are preoccupied with their weight.

In extreme circumstances, the compulsion to lose weight can

'If you're not fuelling your body properly, you'll soon experience extreme fatigue and your running times will slow down'

develop into an eating disorder. The two most recognised are anorexia nervosa and bulimia nervosa. Anorexia nervosa is an extremely restrictive eating behaviour in which the individual restricts food and feels fat despite being 15 per cent or more below an ideal body weight. Bulimia nervosa refers to a cycle of food restriction followed by bingeing and purging.

But there's a third type – disordered eating – which experts think could become a serious problem in the UK. Disordered eating is anything outside of normal eating. Normal eating is when a person eats when they're hungry, stops when they're full and has a varied, balanced diet. But when someone consistently ignores feelings of hunger or fullness, or severely restricts their food choices, they are regarded as having disordered eating. Runners often engage in disordered eating in an attempt to lose weight.

CROSSING THE LINE

Many runners admit to having an addictive nature. Running requires drive, but there's a fine line between self-motivation and obsessiveness. In fact, the personality characteristics needed to become a top athlete are also common in people with eating disorders. These include perfectionism, competitiveness and obsessiveness.

Surveys of elite female runners have found many to be obsessive calorie counters who follow restricted and nutritionally deficient diets, while an American study of 265 recreational female runners found 25 per cent had attitudes to food suggestive of an eating disorder.

Experts believe that, in most cases, disordered eating is a response to an emotional problem. Low self-esteem is a common factor, particularly when combined with poor body image.

WARNING SIGNS

Few people could describe their diet as perfect, but when does eating cross the line from normal to disordered?

One of the most common symptoms is an intense fear of gaining weight. Disordered eaters are preoccupied with food, often fantasising about what they'd like to eat, or feeling guilty about what they've eaten. They often impose strict dietary rules and exercise excessively.

Secret eating is another symptom of disordered eating. Some will eat normal or restrictive meals in public, but may binge when alone, while others skip meals, telling themselves they don't have time to eat.

HEALTH HAZARD

The long-term effect of disordered eating can seriously damage your health. If you're not fuelling your body properly, you'll soon lose energy and experience extreme fatigue. Performance will suffer, your running times will slow down and your aerobic capacity (the ability to take up oxygen during exercise) will reduce. You'll become more susceptible to illness and injury, and recovery time will be longer, as without enough dietary protein to maintain and repair your body, there'll be a loss of lean tissue.

In women, one important cut-off between healthy and unhealthy thinness is the presence of regular periods. If your periods have stopped (secondary amenorrhoea), you risk bone-density loss. Without enough oestrogen to maintain and increase bone mass, the bones get weaker, which may result in premature osteoporosis.

BREAKING THE PATTERN

If you're worried you may be displaying symptoms of disordered eating, the next step is to identify the emotional issues behind your behaviour. You can then learn new ways of coping. Try keeping a food and mood diary for a few weeks, recording what you eat and how you feel as you eat.

You should start choosing a wide variety of foods from each food group, and be realistic about your goal weight – you may be striving to attain a low weight that's inappropriate for your genetic body type. If you have weight to lose, don't crash diet, and seek advice from a dietitian if you're struggling to balance food intake and exercise.

FOR MORE INFORMATION
To find a qualified nutritionist or dietitian, contact www. freelancedietitian.org
For help and support, contact eating disorder charity Beat at www.b-eat.co.uk

ARE YOU A DISORDERED EATER?

Three or more of the following symptoms could be a sign of disordered eating:

▸▸ You constantly think about food.
▸▸ **You often ignore hunger.**
▸▸ You believe you're fat when others insist you're slim.
▸▸ **You often eat past the point of fullness.**
▸▸ You often feel guilty after eating.
▸▸ **You avoid certain foods, even though you want to eat them.**
▸▸ You eat normally with others, but overeat when alone.
▸▸ **You feel stressed or guilty if your normal diet or exercise routine is interrupted.**

THE FOLLOWING WARNING SIGNS COULD INDICATE AN EATING PROBLEM:

▸▸ Unexplained dip in performance.
▸▸ **An obsession with body image and weight.**
▸▸ Constant use of weighing scales.
▸▸ **Missing meals.**
▸▸ Rapid mood swings.
▸▸ **Rapid and significant weight loss.**

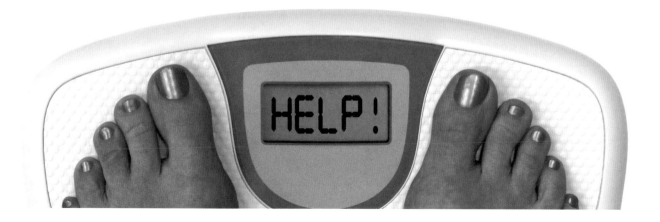

SUPERFOODS
FOR RUNNING

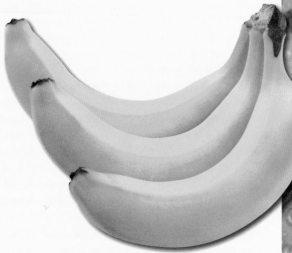

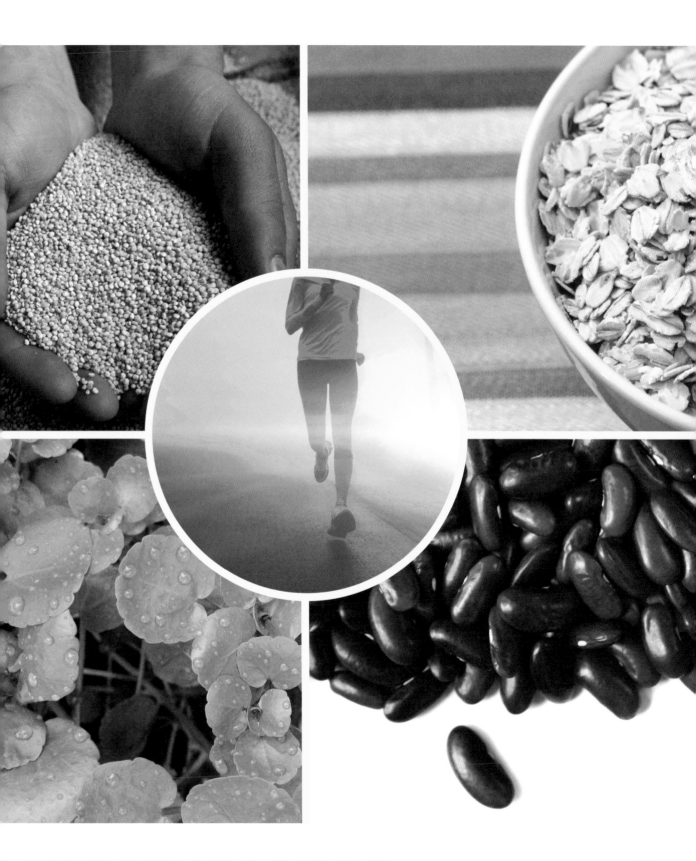

A GUIDE TO
SUPERFOODS

LOOKING FOR HEALTHY OPTIONS TO KEEP YOU FUELLED AND ENERGISED? THEN PILE YOUR PLATE WITH AN ARRAY OF SUPERFOODS. HERE ARE TEN OF THE BEST

While there is no legal definition of a superfood, they are generally considered to be natural foods with an exceptionally high nutrient density including phytonutrients and antioxidants important for health. Superfoods may include ancient foods used by cultures for thousands of years as well as everyday unprocessed natural foods. So if you're looking to boost your health and training, here are our top ten foods to stock up on…

SALMON

Good For: Flexible joints.
Salmon and other smaller oily fish such as sardines and mackerel are packed with anti-inflammatory omega-3 fatty acids, energy boosting CoQ10 and protein to fuel your muscles. A perfect food to help alleviate muscle soreness after long runs and keep joints pain free and flexible. Eat tinned salmon or sardines with the bones for a boost of vitamin D, an important bone-supporting nutrient.
Eat two to three portions (100g per portion) a week.

BERRIES & ACAI

Good For: Recovery.
Naturally energising berries such as strawberries, blueberries, raspberries and cherries are packed with potent antioxidants known as anthocyanins which may help with post exercise recovery and muscle repair. For a real antioxidant hit try acai berries – available as a juice, powder or capsule. Açaí contains ten or more antioxidants than blueberries and 30 times more than red wine. It is also packed with essential fats to combat inflammation. Try adding a spoonful of the powder to a smoothie or stir into yogurt. Aim to eat ½ cup of berries daily.

MACA

Good For: Natural energy.
Known as Peruvian ginseng, maca is a favourite food in South America and regarded as an energy tonic. It is also an adaptogen meaning it can counter the effects of training on the body, balance hormones and improve stamina. Available as a powder, maca is incredibly nutrient dense containing plenty of amino acids, calcium, magnesium, potassium, phosphorus and B vitamins. Try 1-2tsp daily stirred into yogurt, a smoothie or porridge.

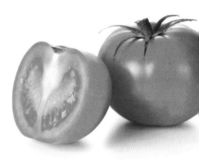

TOMATOES

Good For: Skin protection.
Consuming more lycopene – the carotenoid that makes tomatoes red – may protect your skin from sunburn, ideal for outdoor runners. They are also packed with an array of other energising nutrients including B vitamins, magnesium and potassium. Snack on a handful of cherry

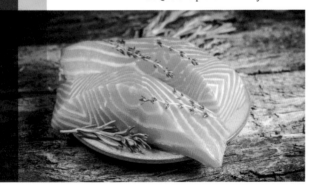

tomatoes, make use of canned tomatoes or drink a small glass of tomato juice 2-3 times a week.

COCONUT WATER AND COCONUT BUTTER

Good For: Endurance and hydration. Coconut butter is a useful source of medium-chain triglycerides (MCT), which are metabolised readily for energy by your liver rather than being stored as fat. This makes it an ideal fuel for long runs. Use as a spread, as a cooking oil or add to a pre-workout smoothie. Coconut water is an excellent hydrating drink – packed with essential electrolytes such as sodium, potassium, magnesium and calcium, which we lose via sweat during exercise. Take a bottle with you on longer runs.

ALMONDS AND OTHER NUTS

Good For: Blood sugar balance. Nuts offer a nutritious package of protein, fibre, and heart-healthy unsaturated fat to keep blood sugar levels balanced and avoid energy dips. Make up a mix with some dried fruit for an ideal nourishing snack during longer running sessions. Almonds are rich in energising iron, B vitamins and protein plus calcium, magnesium and vitamin E – important for muscle recovery. Aim to eat a small handful of nuts daily.

GREEN LEAFY VEGETABLES

Good For: Healthy bones. Broccoli, kale, spinach and other leafy greens are not only packed with energising B vitamins, magnesium and iron to fuel your runs but a great source of bone-supporting nutrients too, including calcium, magnesium and vitamin K. One cup of cooked kale (130g) provides just 36 calories and over 1062mcg vitamin K, which plays an important role in bone health. Aim to eat one to two cupfuls of lightly steamed or raw leafy greens at least two to three times a week.

YOGURT AND KEFIR

Good For: Healthy digestion. Yogurt and kefir provide muscle-friendly protein as well as probiotics that keep your digestive tract healthy and your immune system in top form. Kefir is a cultured milk drink that contains a greater array of probiotic bacteria than yogurt. It also contains conjugated linoleic acid (CLA), which has been shown to help reduce body fat. Try drinking ½ cup kefir daily or natural live yogurt as a healthy snack.

OATS

Good For: Long-lasting energy. Oats are an excellent source of slow releasing carbohydrates and soluble fibre to fuel your runs. They are also packed with immune supporting nutrients including selenium and beta glucans. Consuming slow releasing carbohydrates within 1-2 hours before a long run can help maintain the intensity of training without hunger pangs setting in. Try a bowl of steaming porridge 1-2 hours before a long run. Alternatively, add a couple of spoonfuls of oats to a smoothie.

'Nuts offer a nutritious package of protein, fibre and heart-healthy unsaturated fat, to keep blood sugar levels balanced'

RAW CACAO AND DARK CHOCOLATE

Good For: Mood. If you love chocolate try raw cacao. One of nature's highest dietary sources of magnesium, raw cacao beans and nibs are also rich in iron and an excellent source of dietary fibre. Antioxidant-rich too, cacao beans contain flavonoids, and powerful alkaloid chemicals including theobromine, phenylethylamine and anandamine. These stimulate healthy brain function and feelings that are similar to being in love! So for a quick mood boost, try a handful of cacao nibs or snack on a couple of squares of dark chocolate. Alternatively add a spoonful of raw cacao powder to your favourite smoothie.

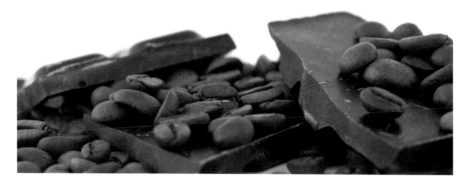

SWEET POTATOES

Despite their name, sweet potatoes are not a type of potato. They aren't even related! They belong to the *Convolvulaceae* plant family. Water spinach, also known as 'morning glory', is the other best-known family member. Originally from Central America, and now grown in warm climates around the world, they've been enjoyed as a nutritious vegetable for more than 5,000 years. Christopher Columbus brought sweet potatoes to Europe after his first voyage to the New World in 1492.

The most common type of sweet potato eaten in the UK has orange flesh, but some varieties have white or even purple flesh. The colour of the flesh reflects the presence of different types of antioxidants.

WHY EAT THEM?

Sweet potatoes are an ideal runner's fuel. Low in fat, they brim with carbohydrates and have a low-glycaemic index (GI), so they slowly release energy-giving glucose into the bloodstream. They pack in essential nutrients, too: vitamin C for a strong immune system; magnesium which helps the body to use energy from food; manganese, important for healthy bones and joints; and beta-carotene (responsible for their orange colour), which the body converts to skin- and eye-friendly vitamin A.

Beta-carotene and vitamin C also work as antioxidants, helping to protect your body's cells – including muscle cells and specialist cells of the immune system – from the potentially damaging effects of free radicals, molecules that can impair tissues. Free radicals are produced naturally by your body as a by-product of daily metabolism, and production is increased by exercise, stress, smoking, poor diet and excess alcohol consumption.

Sweet potatoes are best enjoyed as part of a meal at least two hours before your run. This allows time for your meal to digest and will help provide that slow-release energy so vital for running.

They're also great as part of a balanced post-run meal – their carb content will contribute to refuelling your muscles, ready for the next day.

HOW TO EAT THEM

One medium sweet potato (80g cooked weight) counts as one portion towards the recommended five-a-day fruit and vegetables, and provides around 80 calories – similar to a medium slice of wholegrain bread. Cut into chunks and enjoy boiled, baked or roasted (brushed with a little olive oil) – you can leave the skin on if you like. Also great in a vegetable-based soup, pasta sauce, curry or risotto, or combined with potatoes for an exotic mash. Simply enjoy sweet potatoes as part of a balanced meal as often as you fancy.

'Sweet potatoes
will contribute to
refuelling your
muscles, ready for
the next day'

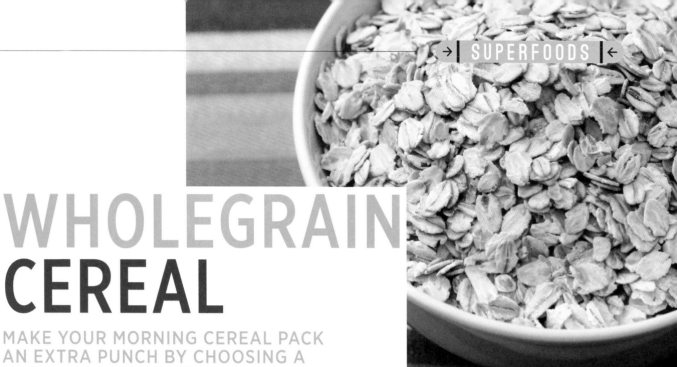

WHOLEGRAIN
CEREAL

MAKE YOUR MORNING CEREAL PACK AN EXTRA PUNCH BY CHOOSING A WHOLEGRAIN VARIETY

WHAT IS IT?

Any variety of breakfast cereal is fine, as long as it's labelled "wholegrain", and "wholegrain cereals" or "whole wheat" is the first ingredient in the ingredients list. Serve with skimmed or semi-skimmed milk.

WHY EAT IT?

Every time you run, you tap into your muscles' energy stores (glycogen). You also increase the natural rate of muscle protein breakdown. Refuelling after running enhances the speed at which your body recovers from these effects of exercise, helps reduce muscle stiffness and helps you to get fitter, faster.

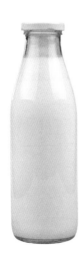

A recent study in the *Journal of the International Society of Sports Nutrition* found that compared with a commercial sports drink, a bowl of wholegrain cereal and skimmed milk was at least as good at promoting muscle refuelling and recovery after two hours of moderately intense exercise. The cereal also helped replenish glycogen in muscles just as well as the carbohydrate-containing sports drink. But cereal had a slight edge on the sports drink when it came to rebuilding muscle protein, no doubt thanks to the amino acids (building blocks of protein) in the milk. This tallies with research highlighting that optimal post-exercise muscle-replenishing snacks combine both carbohydrates and protein.

Wholegrain cereal is also cheaper than sports drinks – and is packed with a wide range of vitamins and minerals. Fortified breakfast cereals provide useful amounts of B vitamins, which allow the body to release energy from food, and iron, to help prevent energy-sapping anaemia. The milk also brims with protein and bone-strengthening calcium. While wholegrain cereal makes a great exercise-recovery snack, a bowl of low-fat, carb-rich cereal is also a good option before you head out for that long run.

HOW TO EAT IT

The study cited above used a large bowl of wholegrain cereal (73g) with 350ml skimmed milk, but a smaller serving would still be beneficial. Refuelling snacks such as this are best eaten within 30 minutes to two hours of finishing your run – and best

'Wholegrain cereal is packed with a wide range of vitamins and minerals'

enjoyed after every running session. And don't forget a drink as well – water is fine. The lightness of this snack can be handy if you find eating difficult after running. If you're using it as a pre-run snack, eat it about two hours beforehand, to ensure your stomach feels comfortable when you run. And don't think cereal is only useful before or after a morning run. It can be a convenient, affordable and tasty running superfood any time of the day. You can also top with some fresh or dried fruit for an extra nutrient boost.

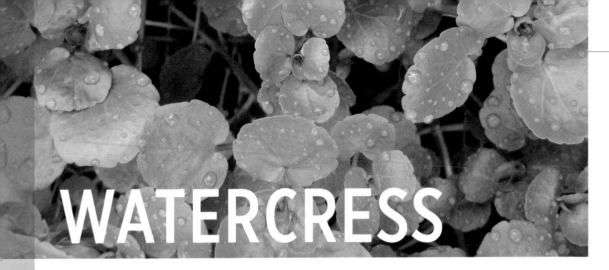

WATERCRESS

INCREASE YOUR IRON INTAKE AND BOOST YOUR IMMUNE SYSTEM WITH THIS UNDER-APPRECIATED RUNNING SUPERFOOD

WHAT IS IT?

Watercress, or *Rorippa nasturtium-aquaticum*, is a member of the cruciferae family and is related to cabbage, Brussels sprouts, broccoli and pak choi.

Believed to have originated in Ancient Greece, and enjoyed widely as a food and remedy throughout the Mediterranean, over the centuries its popularity has spread worldwide. A long-standing British favourite, it had herbal uses in the 1600s and has been grown in spring waters for sale as a vegetable since the 1800s.

In 500BC, Hippocrates, the father of medicine, is said to have located his first hospital close to a stream, to ensure a constant supply of fresh watercress to help treat his patients.

WHY EAT IT?

This superfood brims with essential nutrients, including vitamins A, C and E for healthy skin and a strong immune system, and calcium and vitamin K, both important for blood clotting and bone strength.

It also packs in folic acid and iron, both crucial to build healthy red blood cells, needed for transporting oxygen to help fuel your working muscle cells. Due to menstruation, women of child-bearing age have higher iron needs than men, and a

recent study at the University of Udine in Italy found that 50 per cent of women doing around 11 hours of exercise a week were iron deficient, putting them at risk of fatigue, irritability and poor stamina. The vitamin C in watercress boosts the absorption of its iron content, too – great news for non-meat eaters (iron is better absorbed from meat than vegetable sources).

Watercress also contains lutein, beta-carotene and flavonoids, which, along with vitamins C and E, act as antioxidants. Antioxidants help protect your body's cells, including muscle cells and specialist cells of the immune system, from the potentially damaging effects of free radicals. Production of free radicals is increased during exercise – they're a by-product of using oxygen to produce energy. If left unchecked, damage to cell membranes may worsen post-run muscle soreness. Your body makes its own antioxidants, but when needs are increased, antioxidants from fruit and veg, including watercress, give them a helping hand. Regular training helps boost your body's natural antioxidant defences, too.

Watercress's distinctive peppery taste is thanks to a beneficial plant compound called phenethyl isothiocyanate (PEITC), which in a wide number of scientific studies, including one published in the journal *Carcinogenesis*, has been shown to have a range of anti-cancer properties.

HOW TO EAT IT

Enjoy watercress regularly as part of your balanced, fruit- and veg-rich diet. A portion is a cereal bowl-ful (equivalent to 80g). Watercress is versatile and its unique flavour is great in pasta sauces and stir-fries (toss in at the last minute), baked fish dishes, sandwiches, wraps, mashed potato or mixed with other salad leaves. Watercress can also be used in smoothies – a delicious way to give those tired muscles a post-run antioxidant and carb boost.

PEAR, MELON AND WATERCRESS SMOOTHIE

Cut the flesh of one Galia melon and two pears into bite-sized pieces. Place the fruit, together with 85g watercress, through a juicer and pour into two glasses, stir and enjoy (117 calories, 26g carbohydrate and 1g fat per glass).

'Watercress packs in folic acid and iron, both crucial to build healthy red blood cells'

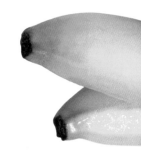

BANANAS

THE ULTIMATE FAST FOOD, BANANAS ARE THE PERFECT FUEL FOR RUNNERS

WHAT ARE THEY?

Originating from South-East Asia, and first cultivated in Papua New Guinea, later Buddhist writings dating from 600BC recorded their presence in India where their convenience took the fancy of Alexander the Great. He initiated their emergence in the Western world. These days, bananas are grown in countries throughout the tropics. Banana plants (bananas don't grow on trees), which are tall and leafy, bear banana fruit hanging down in bunches, and belong to the *Musaceae* plant family, along with 'plantain', a firmer, starchy, non-sweet variety that needs cooking.

WHY EAT THEM?

Bananas are packed with energy-giving carbohydrate, a medium banana contains around 95 calories (the same as 100g of tuna). They also have a low-glycaemic index (GI), meaning their energy is released in a slow and sustained way, ideal for fuelling your running and aiding post-

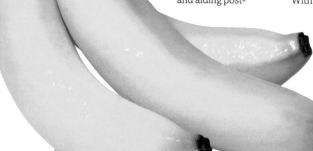

run muscle recovery. A banana counts as one portion towards the recommended five or more portions of fruit and vegetables a day, and brims with cell- and immunity-protecting antioxidants, including vitamin C.

One banana also provides a third of your daily vitamin B6 needs. This vitamin is required to build the mood- and appetite-regulating neurotransmitter (chemical messenger) serotonin. Its ability to help prevent energy-sapping anaemia and regulate blood sugar levels is good news for runners.

HEALTHY CONTENT

Bananas are perhaps best known for their potassium content, a mineral that often goes short in the British diet but is so important, especially for runners. Potassium plays a major role in ensuring normal cell function, proper nerve signals, heart beats and muscle contractions, as well as helping to keep the body hydrated and blood pressure in check.

With all these benefits, snacking on

a banana once or twice a day is no bad thing – it's great as part of a balanced meal, or as a pre- or post-running fuel/refuel snack (think banana smoothie, or banana plus

'One banana provides a third of your daily vitamin B6 needs'

yogurt and a drink). Some people find they can eat them 30 minutes or so before running – others find they need at least an hour's gap to avoid stomach discomfort. As always, you need to test what works best for you in training.

HOW TO EAT THEM

Bananas are so versatile; the ways they can be eaten are only limited by your imagination! Whizzed into smoothies, chopped on cereal or into fruit salad, in a sandwich (plain or toasted) with dates, honey and/or peanut butter, baked, flambéed or fresh and topped with low-fat yogurt or custard, with pancakes, or simply peeled and enjoyed any time. For extra convenience, keep some at work, in a box in your kit bag or even in your handbag (to avoid squashing) or in the fridge at home. Ripe bananas will last longer if stored in the fridge. The skin will go brown but the flesh will still be fine.

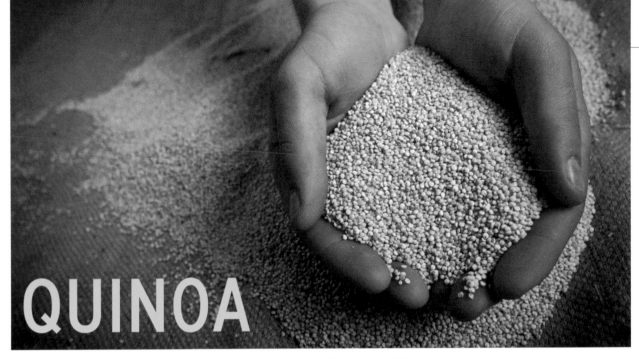

QUINOA

PACKED WITH PROTEIN AND ESSENTIAL MINERALS, THIS SEED IS IDEAL FOR MUSCLE RECOVERY POST-RUN

Botanically known as *Chenopodium quinoa* and pronounced 'keen-wah', quinoa, despite its appearance, is not a grain like wheat or rice, but the seed of a leafy plant related to spinach. It originates from the Andes mountain ranges of Bolivia, Peru and Chile, where it has been an important food for more than 5,000 years. When cooked, it has a spiral-like appearance, with a mild nutty taste and a light, fluffy texture. It's suitable for people on a gluten-free diet and makes a tasty, nutritious alternative to rice, couscous, corn and barley.

WHY EAT IT?

The South American Incas believed this sacred 'mother seed' increased the stamina of their warriors. Modern day nutritional science has revealed quinoa is a good source of balanced protein, similar to the quality of milk protein (good news for vegans), and contains twice as much protein as rice. As well as supporting post-running muscle recovery, protein helps you feel fuller for longer, making

it easier to keep calorie intake – and weight – in check. Quinoa also brims with energy-giving carbohydrates, which are slowly released to provide a steady fuel supply to exercising or refuelling muscles. More good news is that it supplies the key minerals iron (prevents energy-sapping anaemia), bone-friendly magnesium, zinc (for a strong immune system) and potassium (essential for muscle

'Quinoa is a good source of balanced protein'

contraction and keeping the body hydrated), along with folic acid, needed to enable the body to use protein to repair itself, and to prevent anaemia.

Quinoa is best enjoyed as part of a balanced meal at least two hours before you run, to allow time for your meal to digest and to help provide slow-release energy. It's also ideal as

part of a post-run meal – its carb and protein content contributes to refuelling and restoring your muscles. And if you're a runner with a sensitive stomach, quinoa is easy to digest, which could just make it your new best friend.

HOW TO EAT IT

A natural source of fibre, a 50g (before cooking) portion is low in fat and provides 165 calories, similar to two slices of bread. Quinoa is available in major supermarkets and health food shops. Rinse well and boil in plenty of water or vegetable stock until absorbed (around 15 minutes), according to directions on the packet. For a richer flavour, toast quinoa in a dry pan for a minute or two (take care to avoid burning) before cooking. Try quinoa in place of rice, couscous, cracked wheat or barley in soups, stuffed vegetables, pilafs or salads, or as a side dish as an alternative to potatoes, rice or bread. Or use instead of oats in porridge or rice in rice pudding – delicious topped with fresh berries or other fruit, nuts and honey!

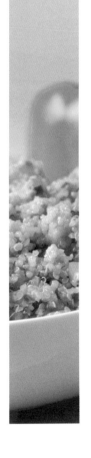

BEETROOT

A RENOWNED APHRODISIAC DURING ROMAN TIMES, THIS SUPERFOOD MAY NOT JUST BE BENEFICIAL FOR YOUR RUNNING PERFORMANCE!

WHAT IS IT?

Beetroot is the red root of the plant species *Beta vulgaris*. Its wild ancestor is sea beet, found along coasts from Britain to the Mediterranean to India. Valued as an aphrodisiac by the Romans, it used to be a white root vegetable – the round red beetroot we know today was not cultivated until the 1500s. It became highly prized in Eastern and Central Europe, especially as an ingredient in the traditional soup, borscht. Its popularity grew in the UK during Victorian times, and it was used in both savoury and sweet dishes.

WHY EAT IT?

Freshly grated or cooked (but not pickled), beetroot brims with folic acid, needed for cell division and building healthy red blood cells, which transport oxygen to help fuel your working muscles. It has been ranked among the top ten most powerful vegetable sources of antioxidants, thanks to antioxidants such as phenolics and betacyanin (which makes it gorgeously red), and it also packs in potassium, an electrolyte lost in sweat while running. Replacing it is a vital part of keeping the body well hydrated. Drinking 500ml (two large glasses) of beetroot juice a day could even help you exercise for 16 per cent longer at the same intensity, according to a study in the *Journal of Applied Physiology*. Scientists think this is due to the nitrate in beetroot, which helps the body use oxygen more efficiently when exercising. The same study also found drinking 500ml of beetroot juice for six days is beneficial for blood pressure levels.

Further support comes from London-based research, which reported a reduction in blood pressure three hours after subjects drank 500ml of beetroot juice.

HOW TO EAT IT

Three baby beetroots or seven slices (fresh or pickled) is equivalent to one of the recommended five-a-day portions of fruit and vegetables. Enjoy beetroot roasted, pickled, steamed, in soup or grated raw into salads or sandwiches. You could try trimming whole beetroot, wrapping in foil and baking until tender. Then simply peel and serve as a hot vegetable, or wait for it to cool, then slice and scatter with goats' cheese and walnuts.

If you have red urine after tucking into beetroot, don't worry. It's a harmless side effect known as 'beeturia' caused by betacyanin passing out in the urine. Thought to affect around one in seven people, it's not clear why it happens, but in some cases it has been linked with a higher risk of being iron deficient. If you also feel tired all the time and find running has become harder work, it's worth seeing your doctor to check your iron and haemoglobin levels.

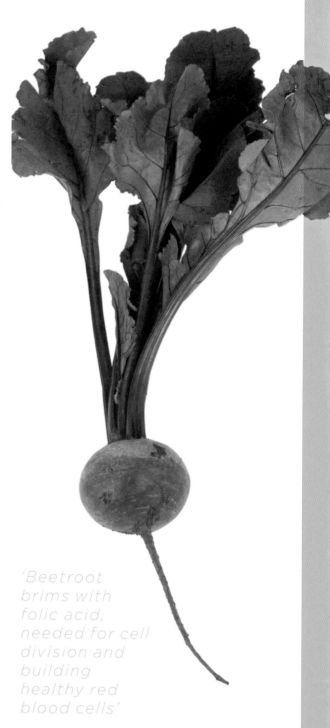

'Beetroot brims with folic acid, needed for cell division and building healthy red blood cells'

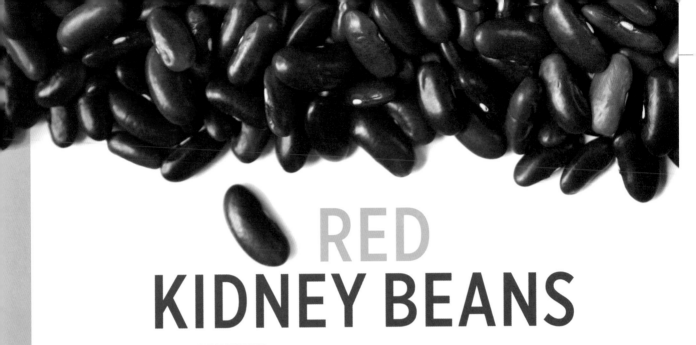

RED KIDNEY BEANS

WHAT ARE THEY?

Originating from Peru, red kidney beans (botanically known as *Phaseolus vulgaris L*) spread throughout South and Central America when used as trade goods. They were introduced into Europe in the 1500s by Spanish explorers returning from their voyages to the New World. Later, Spanish and Portuguese traders acquainted Africa

'Red kidney beans are brilliant for vitamin B1, needed to release the energy stored in carbohydrate'

and Asia with kidney beans. As red kidney and other beans are an easily stored, inexpensive and nutritious form of protein, they have become part of many different diets throughout the world.

WHY EAT THEM?

Kidney beans are naturally low in fat and brim with muscle-fuelling carbohydrate. They also have a low glycaemic index (GI), meaning they provide a slow, steady release of energy-giving glucose into the bloodstream. Red kidney beans rank

IT MAY BE A HUMBLE BEAN, BUT IT CERTAINLY PACKS A PUNCH WHEN IT COMES TO PROTECTING YOUR HEALTH AND FUELLING YOUR RUNNING!

third in a top-20 list of antioxidant-rich foods, according to a study by the United States Department of Agriculture (USDA), and in a large American study of almost 10,000 men and women, those who ate kidney beans and other pulses four or more times a week had a 22 per cent lower risk of coronary heart disease and an 11 per cent lower risk of heart attack and stroke, compared with infrequent consumers. Kidney beans contain soluble fibre, which absorbs water in the digestive system to form a gel, helping to keep appetite and cholesterol levels in check. Soluble fibre, along with protective antioxidants, helps explain kidney beans' heart-health benefits. Eating kidney beans or other beans and lentils at least twice a week lowers the risk of breast cancer by a third, according to a study of the diet, lifestyle and health of more than 90,000 American women. Again, the beans' fibre and antioxidant content are believed to play key health-

protecting roles. Kidney beans are brilliant for vitamin B1, needed to release the energy stored in carbohydrate, your body's favourite fuel. Vitamin B1 is also essential for healthy nerve and heart function.

HOW TO EAT THEM

Three heaped tablespoons of kidney beans count towards your recommended five-a-day portions of fruit and vegetables. The canned variety are convenient and nutritious. If preparing your own, be sure to follow the instructions on the pack when soaking (to reduce any flatulence side effects!) and cooking dried beans. A good source of protein and iron, kidney beans are a healthy vegetarian alternative to meat. Enjoy in vegetable chilli or casseroles, hearty soups, salads, tacos or wraps (stir-fry with vegetables), patties, or as a bean dip. You can use alongside small portions of meat, in classic dishes such as chilli con carne.

CHOCOLATE MILK

NOT JUST A TASTY TREAT, THIS SUPERFOOD PACKS THE
PERFECT POST-RUN CARBOHYDRATE AND PROTEIN PUNCH

WHAT IS IT?

Hurrah for chocolate milk! This delicious, slightly indulgent superfood serves up a host of research-backed performance benefits (it wasn't spotted in the hands of athletes at the London Olympics for nothing!). If you prefer your milk plain or flavoured in other ways, that's fine too – but always opt for low-fat varieties. As well as being nutritious, the balance of protein, carbohydrate, minerals and water in plain and flavoured milk appear to make it a useful way to refuel and restore after running. Here's the low-down…

WHY DRINK IT?

Chocolate milk has a low glycaemic index (GI), providing slow-release energy, and its protein content helps promote satiety (helping you feel fuller for longer). It's rich in bone-friendly calcium, a mineral also essential for muscle and nerve function, and normal digestion. A 200ml glass of low-fat chocolate (or plain or flavoured) milk provides more than a quarter of the daily recommended intake. Chocolate milk's carbohydrate (from lactose, the natural milk sugar, plus added sugars) and protein content makes it an ideal post-exercise drink for refuelling glycogen stores and optimising muscle repair.

Two recent studies from the University of Connecticut looked specifically at chocolate milk's role for runners. Those who drank 450ml of low-fat chocolate milk after a 45-minute run had better measures of muscle protein repair and glycogen content than those who had 450ml of a calorie-matched, carbohydrate-only drink. It might just boost your performance during your next run, too. Research from the University of Texas found that drinking fat-free chocolate milk, compared with a placebo or carbohydrate drink of similar calorific value, after high-intensity cycling resulted in better trial times in a 40K ride four hours later. Milk is a good way to rehydrate after running by efficiently replacing lost fluid, thanks to its water and electrolyte (minerals such as potassium, chloride and sodium) content. In a study from Loughborough University, plain, low-fat milk even outperformed water and sports drinks, by having more beneficial effects on urine output after exercise. Chocolate milk is also great for riboflavin (vitamin B2), which allows the body to release the energy stored in food, and supports healthy skin and vision.

HOW TO DRINK IT

Most studies use around 450 to 500ml chocolate milk to test its effectiveness, but just one glass (plain or flavoured) can be nutritionally beneficial. Make your own chocolate milk at home using skimmed milk and a chocolate drink powder. If you buy it ready-made, choose brands labelled "low fat". Remember to check and compare products for calorie content. Low-fat chocolate milk typically provides around 125 to 140 calories per 200ml glass.

'Chocolate milk's carbohydrate and protein content makes it an ideal post-exercise drink for refuelling glycogen stores and optimising muscle repair'

RECIPES FOR RUNNERS

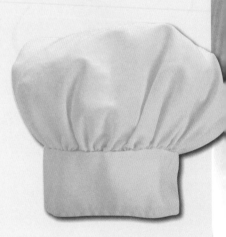

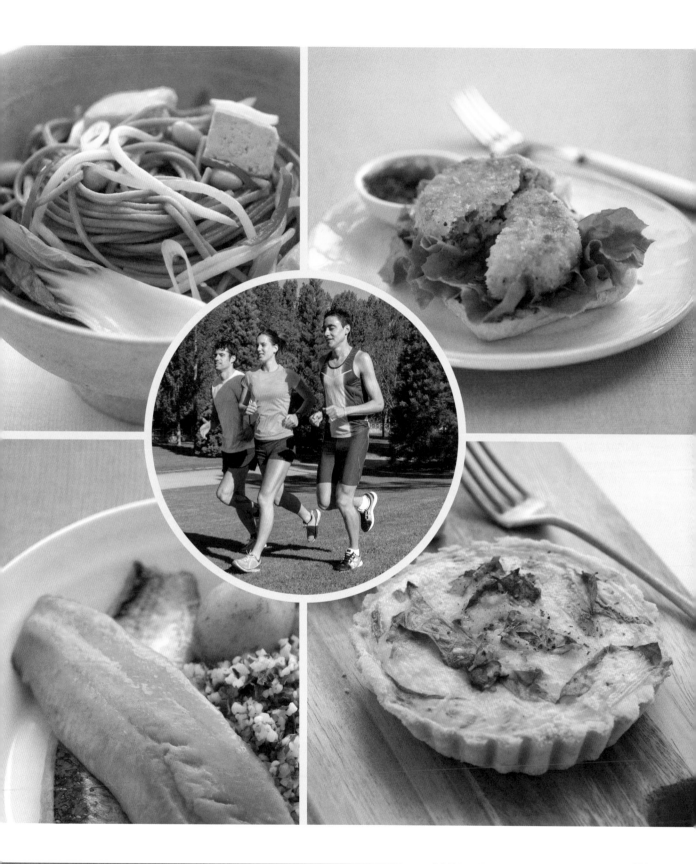

SOBA NOODLES WITH TOFU

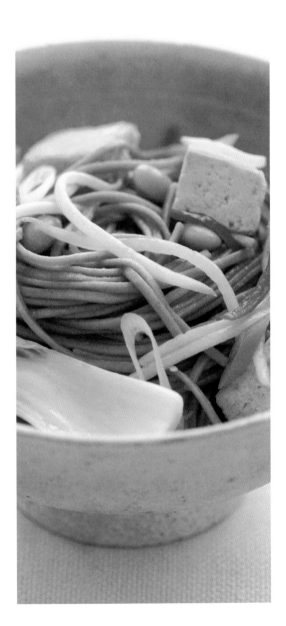

TIP: *To turn this into a meat or fish dish, use chicken or king prawns as an alternative*

KEEP YOUR BLOOD SUGAR LEVELS STABLE THROUGHOUT YOUR RUN WITH THIS DELICIOUS RECIPE

PREPARATION
Serves: 2
Preparation: 10 minutes
Cooking: 10 minutes

INGREDIENTS
- 1tbsp vegetable oil
- 3cm piece of ginger, cut into matchsticks
- ½ red chilli, deseeded and sliced
- 250g firm tofu, cubed
- 2tbsp light soy sauce
- 1tbsp Chinese rice wine
- 200g buckwheat soba noodles
- 100g bean sprouts
- 1 pak choi, core and outer leaves removed
- 50g edamame beans, defrosted
- 1 spring onion, sliced

METHOD:
1: Place the wok over a medium heat, add the oil, ginger and chilli and cook for a few minutes. Carefully add the tofu and cook all sides until golden, then pour the soy sauce and Chinese rice wine into the wok and mix well.

2: Meanwhile, soak the soba noodles in boiling water for five minutes or until soft. Drain and rinse, then add to the wok with the bean sprouts, pak choi leaves and edamame beans.

3: Toss all ingredients together. Check the seasoning and add more soy sauce if required.

4: Serve noodles in a bowl, and garnish with slices of spring onion.

RUNNING BENEFITS
This carbohydrate-rich dish will provide plenty of slow-release carbohydrates, making it ideal to eat two to two-and-a-half hours before your run. Buckwheat is energising and nutritious, supplying plenty of magnesium to relax blood vessels and improve nutrient delivery. It's also rich in iron, which assists with oxygen delivery to the working muscles.

NUTRITION INFORMATION (PER PERSON)
433 calories; 18g protein; 67g carbohydrate; 12.1g fat (4.25g polyunsaturated, 3.9g monounsaturated, 1.3g saturated); 2.4g fibre

....

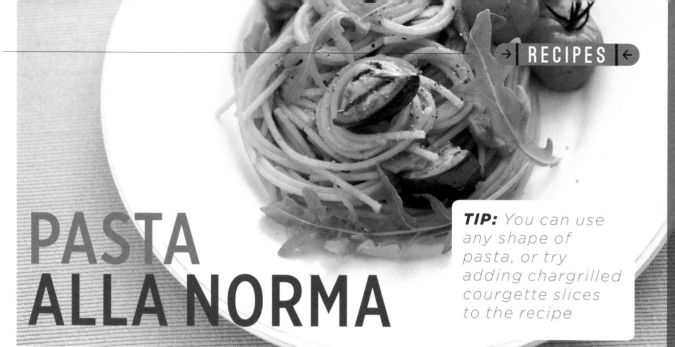

PASTA ALLA NORMA

TIP: *You can use any shape of pasta, or try adding chargrilled courgette slices to the recipe*

BOOST IMMUNITY WITH THIS DELICIOUS SPAGHETTI, AUBERGINE AND TOMATO DISH

PREPARATION
Serves: 2
Preparation: 15 minutes
Cooking: 1 hour 10 minutes

INGREDIENTS
- 1tsp olive oil
- 1 onion, chopped
- 2 garlic cloves, thinly sliced
- 5 ripe tomatoes, deseeded and chopped
- 1 tsp brown sugar
- 150ml water
- 1 tbsp sundried tomato paste
- 1 aubergine, cubed
- 1tsp olive oil
- 6 cherry tomatoes (optional garnish)
- 200g wholegrain spaghetti, cooked
- Salt and black pepper
- 75g rocket leaves, washed
- 50g parmesan, grated (optional)

METHOD:
1. In a large saucepan, heat the oil, add the onion and cook until soft and translucent. Add the garlic and cook for another minute. Tip in the tomatoes, sugar, water and sundried tomato paste. Give the pan a good stir and leave on a simmering heat for 45 minutes. Check regularly and stir.

2. Place the cubed aubergine into a bowl and coat in olive oil. Heat a griddle pan until hot, then carefully griddle each side of the aubergine until chargrilled lines appear and the aubergine is cooked through. Put to one side.

3. Preheat the oven to 190C/180C fan oven/gas mark 5. Place the cherry tomatoes on a baking sheet, drizzle with a splash of olive oil and roast for 15 minutes. Remove from the oven and put to one side.

4. Cook the pasta as per instructions on the packet, then drain and keep warm.

5. Meanwhile, using a hand blender, pulse the tomato sauce until smooth.

Stir in the aubergine and taste. Season with salt and black pepper.

6. Mix the cooked pasta into the tomato and aubergine sauce, sprinkle with Parmesan (if using) and serve with rocket leaves and roasted cherry tomatoes on the side.

RUNNING BENEFITS
This vegetarian fuel-up meal provides plenty of lycopene, a powerful antioxidant that reduces the damage caused by excessive oxygen molecules in the body. With your recommended nutrient intake for vitamin C in one serving and plenty of vitamin A, this dish provides fantastic support for the immune system, too. The wholegrain pasta provides slow-release energy, making it a perfect pre-run meal for two to two-and-a-half hours before your race.

NUTRITION INFORMATION (PER PERSON)
445.5 calories; 18g protein; 82.5g carbohydrate; 7g fat (2.26g polyunsaturated, 2.75g monounsaturated, 1.2g saturated); 14.5g fibre

PERFECT JACKET POTATO WITH HOMEMADE COLESLAW

TUCK INTO THESE FAST-DIGESTING CARBS BEFORE YOUR RUN FOR AN EXTRA SURGE OF POWER

PREPARATION

Serves: 4
Preparation: 15 minutes
Cooking: 1 hour

INGREDIENTS

» 4 jacket potatoes
» 2tbsp olive oil
» Pinch of sea salt
» ¼ white cabbage, finely sliced
» ½ celeriac, peeled and finely sliced
» 1 red onion, finely sliced
» 1 carrot, grated
» 75ml goats' milk live organic yogurt
» 1tsp grainy mustard
» Cracked black pepper
» Handful of chives, chopped

METHOD

1. Preheat the oven to 200C/190C fan oven/gas mark 6. Place the potatoes in a roasting tin, brush each one with olive oil and sprinkle with sea salt. This will make the skins crispy. Cook in the oven for one hour.

2. In the meantime, make the coleslaw. Place all the vegetable ingredients in a large bowl and toss. Next, add the goats' yogurt and grainy mustard, and combine well. Season with black pepper and add the chopped chives.

RUNNING BENEFITS

This recipe is perfect to fuel you for a run, with fast-digesting carbohydrate in the jacket potato and a small amount of protein to aid transport of this fuel to the muscles. Rich in the minerals zinc and iron, plus vitamins A and C, it's a great way to bolster your immune system prior to an event and it tastes great.

NUTRITIONAL INFORMATION (PER PERSON)

338.5 calories; 9.3g protein; 62g carbohydrate; 6.8g fat (0.8g polyunsaturated, 4.5g monounsaturated, 1.4g saturated)

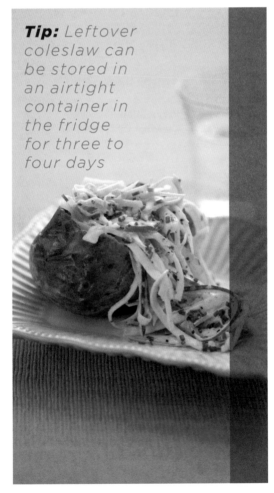

Tip: Leftover coleslaw can be stored in an airtight container in the fridge for three to four days

SEARED TUNA WITH LENTILS AND TOMATOES

FUEL YOUR MUSCLES WITH THE SLOW-RELEASE CARBS FOUND IN LENTILS

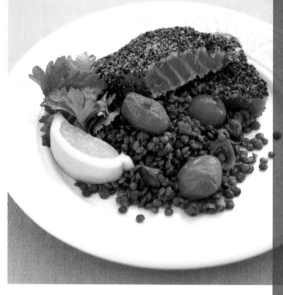

TIP: *If you'd prefer rare tuna steaks, grill on a high heat for about one minute on each side*

PREPARATION
Serves: 2
Preparation: 10 minutes
Cooking: 25 minutes

INGREDIENTS
- 150g cherry tomatoes
- 1tbsp olive oil
- 500ml chicken stock
- 200g lentils
- 1tbsp olive oil
- 1 red onion, finely diced
- 2 garlic cloves, finely diced
- ½ tsp ground cumin
- 30g crushed black pepper
- 2 x 115g tuna steaks
- Juice of 1 lemon

METHOD
1. Preheat the oven to 190C/170C fan oven/gas mark 5. Place the tomatoes in a roasting tin with a dash of oil and roast in the oven for 15 minutes.

2. In a hot frying pan, add another a splash of oil, then fry the red onion until soft. Add the garlic and cumin, and cook for a further minute. Place to one side. Next, pour the chicken stock into a saucepan, add the lentils and cook until soft, then drain and mix with the red onion.

3. Tip the black pepper onto a saucer and coat both sides of the tuna steaks. In a hot pan, add the remaining oil and sear each side of the tuna steaks for three to four minutes (to cook them medium rare).

4. To serve, slice the tuna and serve on a bed of lentils with the roasted tomatoes and a drizzle of lemon juice.

RUNNING BENEFITS
This iron- and zinc-rich dish provides perfect support for your immune system the night before a race, while the slow-release carbohydrates in the lentils will help to fill up your energy stores for the next morning's run, and the protein in the tuna will support muscle repair. It's rich in B vitamins too, which helps with energy transportation. Tuna and lentils contain tryptophan, an amino acid that raises serotonin levels, so this meal should leave you relaxed and ready for a good night's sleep prior to your race.

NUTRITIONAL INFORMATION (PER PERSON)
504.2 calories; 43.5g protein; 55g carbohydrate; 12.2g fat (5.1g polyunsaturated, 5.6g monounsaturated, 1.6g saturated); 12g fibre

SPINACH AND CHEESE TARTLETS WITH BROAD BEAN, FETA AND OLIVE SALAD

INDULGE IN THESE DELICIOUS MINERAL-RICH TREATS

PREPARATION

Serves: 2
Preparation: 20 minutes, plus 30 minutes for chilling
Cooking: 40 minutes

INGREDIENTS

- ▸▸ 170g ready-rolled shortcrust pastry
- ▸▸ 2 free range eggs
- ▸▸ 80ml semi-skimmed milk
- ▸▸ 50g spinach, wilted
- ▸▸ 50g cheddar cheese, grated
- ▸▸ Salt and black pepper

Salad
- ▸▸ 100g broad beans, podded
- ▸▸ 50g feta
- ▸▸ 75g black olives
- ▸▸ 1tbsp extra virgin olive oil
- ▸▸ 1tbsp lemon juice
- ▸▸ Salt and black pepper
- ▸▸ Egg wash and flour for dusting

METHOD:

1. Preheat the oven to 200C/190C fan oven/gas mark 6. Lightly flour the work surface and then place the pastry on top. Use a rolling pin, roll to 5mm thick. Take two mini tart cases (approximately 10cm in diameter) and grease with a little melted butter.

2. Cut two pieces of pastry and line each tart case. Place the cases in the fridge for 30 minutes to chill. After this, line them with greaseproof paper and fill with beans. Bake in the preheated oven for ten minutes, then remove the beans and paper. Use a fork to prick the base and then egg wash the pastry case. Return to the oven and continue to bake for five minutes or until the pastry is golden. Cool each tart case on a wire rack.

3. Make the filling by whisking the eggs in a jug with the milk. Add the wilted spinach and grated cheese, and mix well. Season with salt and pepper. Pour the filling into the tart cases and return to the oven at 180C/170C fan oven/gas mark 4 for 12 to 15 minutes.

4. In a medium bowl, make the salad by mixing the broad beans with the feta and olives. Pour over the olive oil and lemon juice, and toss well. Season to taste. Serve the tarts warm or cold with the salad.

NUTRITIONAL INFORMATION (PER PERSON)

TARTLETS
350.8 calories; 18.5g protein; 38g carbohydrate; 13.75g fat (1.43g polyunsaturated, 5.08g monounsaturated, 7.4g saturated); 2.14g fibre

SALAD
165.3 calories; 7g protein; 4.05g carbohydrate; 13.45g fat (1.34g polyunsaturated, 7.23g monounsaturated, 4.9g saturated); 4.14g fibre.

RUNNING BENEFITS

Packed with good fats and fibre, and providing one quarter of the daily requirement of both zinc and iron, plus a healthy dose of selenium, these tasty tartlet treats make a great mineral-rich refuelling option. With the broad beans providing fibre too, you'll be over halfway to meeting your daily requirements.

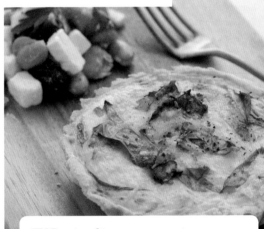

TIP: *Leftover pastry can be carefully wrapped up and placed in the freezer for another time*

REGISTER TODAY FOR THE MEN'S RUNNING E-NEWSLETTER

With our features, forums and exclusive competitions, the *Men's Running* online community is the place for you!

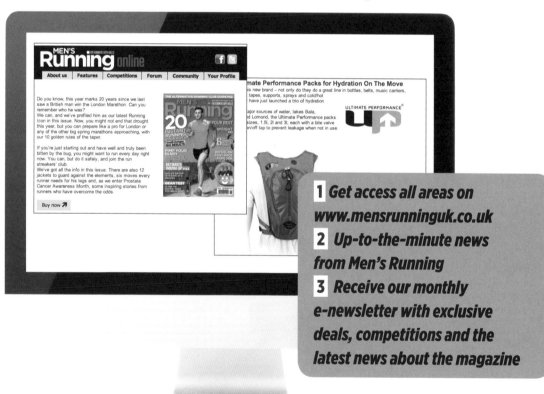

1 *Get access all areas on www.mensrunninguk.co.uk*

2 *Up-to-the-minute news from Men's Running*

3 *Receive our monthly e-newsletter with exclusive deals, competitions and the latest news about the magazine*

Register today!

To enjoy all the best features of the website, follow our fast, simple registration process. You'll be able to access new areas of the site and can receive our free newsletter too

www.mensrunninguk.co.uk

OUR PROMISE – we will never sell or rent your details to third parties

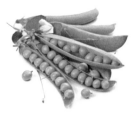

ROASTED BUTTERNUT SQUASH WITH SAUSAGES, PEAS AND QUINOA

THIS SUPER-EASY SUPPER IS PERFECT AFTER A LONG RACE

PREPARATION

Serves: 4
Preparation: 10 minutes
Cooking: 30 minutes

INGREDIENTS

- 1 butternut squash, skin on, chopped into wedges, seeds removed
- 8 Cumberland sausages
- 1tbsp olive oil
- 3 sprigs thyme
- Sea salt
- 120g peas
- 60g quinoa
- 4tsp light cream cheese
- Black pepper

METHOD

1. Preheat the oven to 190C/170C fan oven/gas mark 5.

2. Place the butternut squash and sausages into a roasting tin and drizzle with olive oil. Add the thyme and a sprinkling of sea salt. Place in the oven and roast for 30 minutes, or until the sausages are cooked through and the butternut squash is tender.

3. Meanwhile, cook the peas in boiling water and cook the quinoa as instructed on the pack. Drain the peas and mix with the quinoa.

4. Place wedges of butternut squash and sausages on a bed of peas and quinoa, and add a teaspoon of cream cheese. Season with black pepper and serve immediately.

RUNNING BENEFITS

Increased oxygen use during running leads to the production of oxidants (free radicals). These occur naturally in the body, but too many can damage the body's cells, so this antioxidant- and beta carotene-rich dish is a great choice post-run. Packed with anti-inflammatory beta-carotene, it's also a comforting and tasty recovery option after a longer race, such as a half marathon.

NUTRITIONAL INFORMATION (PER PERSON)

456 calories; 23.4g protein; 32g carbohydrate; 27g fat (4.1g polyunsaturated, 11.8g monounsaturated, 9g saturated); 3.9g fibre

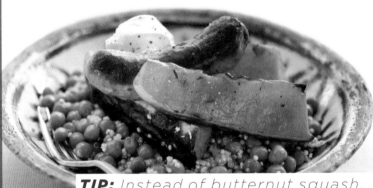

TIP: *Instead of butternut squash, try roasted sweet potatoes*

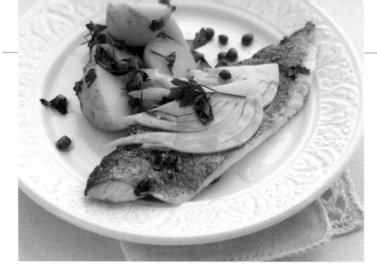

SEA BASS WITH FENNEL AND CAPERS

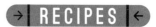

SOOTHE ACHING MUSCLES WITH A MEAL RICH IN ANTI-INFLAMMATORY INGREDIENTS

PREPARATION
Serves: 2
Preparation: 10 minutes
Cooking: 15 minutes

INGREDIENTS
For the fish
- 2 sea bass fillets, pinboned
- ½ fennel bulb, thinly sliced
- 1tsp capers, rinsed
- 1tbsp olive oil
- 1tbsp parsley, chopped
- Sea salt

For the potato salad
- 200g new potatoes
- 1tsp butter
- 1tbsp capers, rinsed and chopped
- 2tbsp parsley, chopped
- 1tsp dill, chopped
- Salt and black pepper

METHOD
1. Preheat the oven to 200C/190C fan oven/gas mark 6. Lay a large piece of tin foil on the work surface and place the two fillets in the middle of the foil, skin-side up. Score the skin of the fish three times and rub a little salt over the skin. Place the fennel slices on the fish, add the capers, drizzle with olive oil and add a scattering of parsley.

2. Fold the tin foil to make a parcel and place on a baking sheet. Put into the preheated oven and cook for 12 to 15 minutes.

3. In the meantime, cook the potatoes to tender and then slice in half. Place in a bowl and toss with the butter, capers and herbs, and season well with salt and pepper.

4. Carefully unwrap the foil parcel and serve the sea bass fillets with the warm potato salad.

RUNNING BENEFITS
This low-fat healthy dish provides plenty of filling lean protein, to support the body's repair process, along with plenty of good fats, to support a healthy immune system. The capers in this dish also contain two bioflavanoids – rutin and quercetin – known to have strong anti-inflammatory benefits.

> **TIP:** Sea bream also works well in this recipe

NUTRITIONAL INFORMATION (PER PERSON)
243 calories; 21.7g protein; 19g carbohydrate; 8.98g fat (1.24g polyunsaturated, 5.14g monounsaturated, 2.6g saturated); 2.49g fibre

TURKEY AND APPLE BURGERS

THESE LOW-GI BURGERS HAVE A HINT OF ANTI-INFLAMMATORY CHILLI TO SOOTHE ACHING LEGS

PREPARATION
Serves: 4
Preparation: 15 minutes, plus 30 minutes for chilling
Cooking: 10 to 15 minutes (chilli relish, 40 minutes)

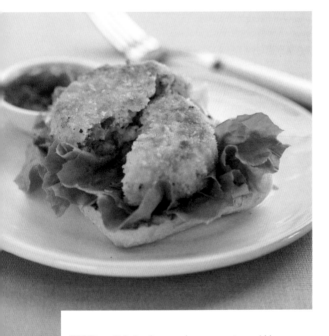

TIP: *Chicken breast will taste equally delicious*

INGREDIENTS
For the chilli relish
- 1tsp olive oil
- ½ red onion, finely diced
- 1 red chilli, finely chopped
- 2 garlic cloves, thinly sliced
- 4 tomatoes, chopped
- 1tbsp balsamic vinegar
- 1tbsp honey
- Pinch of salt and pepper

For the burgers
- 1 celery stick, roughly chopped
- ½ red chilli, deseeded, chopped
- 300g free-range turkey breast
- 1 red apple, cored
- Handful of coriander leaves
- 2tbsp dried breadcrumbs
- Juice from half a lime
- 1 egg, lightly whisked
- Flour for dusting
- Panko (Japanese) breadcrumbs
- 2tbsp vegetable oil, for frying
- 4 ciabatta rolls, toasted
- ¼ green lettuce, torn

METHOD
1. First, make the chilli relish. In a saucepan, add the oil and red onion, and cook until soft and translucent. Next, add the chilli and garlic, and cook for another minute. Tip in the tomatoes and stir.

2. Add the balsamic vinegar and honey, stir again and leave to simmer for 40 minutes, occasionally stirring.

3. When the chilli relish is cooled, put into a sterilised jar with a lid and store in a cool, dark place. Once open, store in the fridge.

4. To make the turkey apple burgers, place the celery, chilli, turkey breast, apple and coriander in a food processor and pulse five or six times. Add the breadcrumbs and lime juice, and season well with salt and black pepper. Pulse again, then tip the mixture into a bowl. Cover with cling film and chill for 30 minutes.

5. Preheat the oven to 190C/170C fan oven/gas mark 5. Take the turkey mix and form four equal-sized burgers and place on a tray.

6. Take three plates: put the seasoned flour on one, lightly whisked egg on the other and panko breadcrumbs on the third. Dust the turkey burgers with seasoned flour and then dip in the egg wash and coat in the breadcrumbs.

7. In a large hot frying pan, add the vegetable oil and turkey burgers, and cook until the breadcrumbs are nice and golden on all sides. Then place into the preheated oven for ten minutes or until cooked.

RUNNING BENEFITS
These tasty turkey burgers deliver a fabulous serving of low-fat protein and low-GI carbohydrate, plus plenty of mood-regulating zinc.

NUTRITIONAL INFORMATION
415 calories; 35.5g protein; 44.9g carbohydrate; 11.6g fat (5.3g polyunsaturated, 9.5g monounsaturated, 4.9g saturated); 7.5g fibre.

CHICKEN CASSEROLE WITH HARICOT BEANS AND TARRAGON

A PROTEIN-RICH STEW TO AID MUSCLE REPAIR AFTER YOUR RUN

PREPARATION

Serves: 4
Preparation: 15 minutes
Cooking: 40-45 minutes

INGREDIENTS

- 4tbsp olive oil
- 5tbsp flour, seasoned
- 4 chicken thighs, skin on
- 4 chicken legs, skin on
- 170g pancetta, cubed
- 1 stick of celery, diced
- 1 carrot, diced
- 1 onion, diced
- 1 garlic clove, chopped
- 1 bay leaf
- 200ml dry white wine
- 700ml chicken stock, warmed
- 1 tin haricot beans, drained
- Handful tarragon leaves, chopped
- Salt and pepper
- 400g new baby potatoes, cooked
- 1 broccoli head, cut into florets and steamed

METHOD

1. Preheat the oven to 180C/160C fan oven/gas mark 4. Add half the olive oil to a large cast-iron casserole dish and heat on the hob. Dust the chicken with the seasoned flour, shake off any excess, add to the dish and brown on all sides. Remove and set aside.

2. Add the remaining olive oil to the casserole dish, add the pancetta and fry until golden. Next, add the celery, carrot and onion, and cook until soft, but not browned. Add the garlic and bay leaf and cook for another minute.

3. Next, pour in the white wine and cook until the liquid reduces by half. Return the chicken to the casserole dish and pour over the chicken stock. Make sure it's just enough to cover the chicken. If not, add some water. Bring to the boil, place a lid over the dish and bake in the oven for 30-40 minutes, or until the chicken is tender.

4. Remove the casserole from the oven and place on the hob over a high heat. Add the beans and reduce the liquid until it has the consistency of a sauce. Add the chopped tarragon and season with salt and pepper.

5. Serve with new potatoes and steamed broccoli on the side.

NUTRITIONAL INFORMATION (PER PERSON)

595.5 calories; 35.3g protein; 45.7g carbohydrate ; 25.8g fat (4.3g polyunsaturated, 15.3g monounsaturated, 6.3g saturated) 6.3g fibre

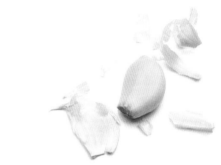

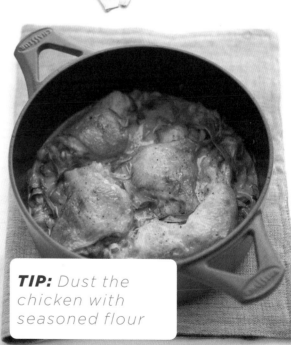

TIP: *Dust the chicken with seasoned flour*

SMOKED KIPPERS WITH BULGAR WHEAT, PARSLEY & MINT SALAD

BOOST YOUR OMEGA 3 INTAKE WITH THIS SUPER-QUICK SUPPER

PREPARATION

Serves: 2
Preparation: 15 minutes
Cooking: 2 minutes

INGREDIENTS

- 100g bulgar wheat
- 1tbsp olive oil
- 200ml boiling water
- 300g Jersey Royals
- 2 mint leaves
- 1 bunch parsley, finely chopped
- 25g mint, chopped
- Juice of one lemon
- Salt and black pepper
- 1tsp butter
- 2 smoked kipper fillets

METHOD

1. Put the bulgar wheat into a heat-proof bowl, pour over the olive oil and stir through. Add boiling water, then cover tightly with cling film and leave to stand for 15 minutes until the liquid has absorbed.

2. In the meantime, wash the Jersey Royals, place in a pan and cover with cold water and the mint leaves. Cook until tender, strain and return to the pan.

3. Return to the bulgar wheat and use a fork to fluff it up, then transfer to a clean bowl. Add the chopped parsley and mint, and toss together. Lastly, add the lemon juice and season with salt and pepper.

4. Melt one teaspoon of butter in a medium frying pan, add the kipper fillets and warm through on both sides.

5. Serve the kippers on a bed of bulgar wheat salad, with the Jersey Royals on the side.

RUNNING BENEFITS

Packed full of healthy fats to support immunity and reduce inflammation from training, this delicious meal also delivers 25mcg of vitamin D, to maintain strong bones. As if that were not enough, kippers also contain phosphorus, potassium, iron and zinc. This is a fabulous dish for boosting your mood and immune system.

NUTRITIONAL INFORMATION (PER PERSON)

575 calories; 33.4g protein; 65.5g carbohydrate; 19.5g fat (3.2g polyunsaturated, 11g monounsaturated, 5g saturated); 1.8g fibre

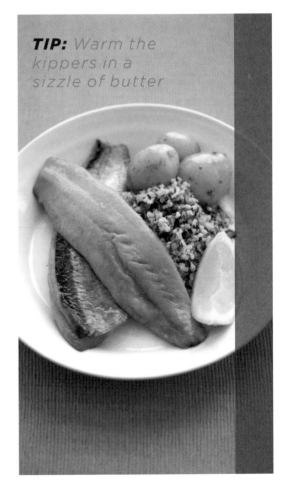

TIP: *Warm the kippers in a sizzle of butter*

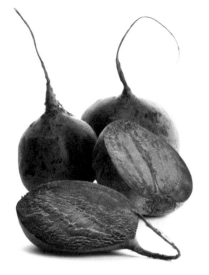

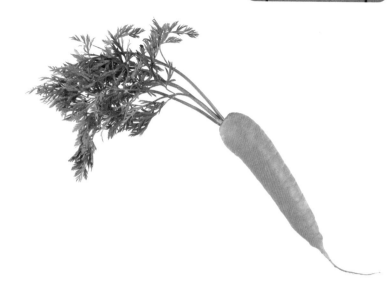

BEETROOT AND CARROT JUICE

BOOST YOUR VITAMIN AND MINERAL INTAKE WITH THIS TASTY VEGGIE JUICE

PREPARATION
Serves: 2
Preparation: 10 minutes

INGREDIENTS
▸▸ 2 raw beetroots, peeled and cut into wedges
▸▸ 3 carrots, peeled
▸▸ 2 conference pears, peeled and cored

METHOD
1. Feed the beetroots, carrots and pears through a juicer and stir well. Pour into chilled glasses and serve.

RUNNING BENEFITS
This is a perfect fibre-rich juice, with the carrots also providing plenty of beta-carotene, potassium, and vitamins C and E. With an added hit of iron, folic acid and vitamin B6 from the beetroot, this juice delivers a concoction of vitamins and minerals to support your health.

NUTRITIONAL INFORMATION (PER PERSON)
150.5 calories; 1.83g protein; 35g carbohydrate; 0.4g fat (0.28g polyunsaturated, 0g monounsaturated, 0.12g saturated); 7.63g fibre

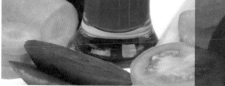

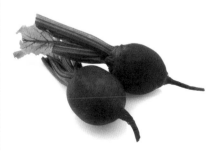

TOMATO, APPLE AND CELERY JUICE

WAKE UP TO A REFRESHING, ANTIOXIDANT-RICH SMOOTHIE. DELICIOUS!

PREPARATION
Serves: 2
Preparation: 10 minutes

INGREDIENTS
▸▸ 500g ripe tomatoes, roughly chopped
▸▸ 2 celery sticks, roughly chopped (plus extra for garnishing)
▸▸ 50ml apple juice
▸▸ 1tsp Worcestershire sauce
▸▸ Few drops Tabasco sauce
▸▸ 1tbsp lime juice
▸▸ Pinch celery salt

METHOD
1. Juice the tomatoes and celery, then pour into a jug. Add the apple juice, Worcestershire sauce, Tabasco sauce, lime juice and celery salt and stir well. Pour over ice and add a leafy stick of celery.

RUNNING BENEFITS
This cleansing, antioxidant-rich juice will stimulate your metabolic rate, making it perfect for a morning pick-you-up.

NUTRITIONAL INFORMATION (PER PERSON)
56 calories; 2g protein; 11g carbohydrate; 0.9g fat; (0.6g polyunsaturated, 0.3g monounsaturated, trace saturated); 2.8g fibre

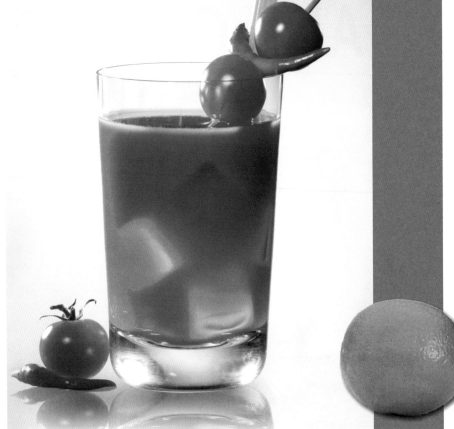

CARROT AND MELON JUICE

GIVE YOUR IMMUNE SYSTEM A KICK-START WITH THIS ULTRA-REFRESHING DRINK

PREPARATION

Serves: 2
Preparation: 5 minutes

INGREDIENTS

» 300g fresh carrots
» 1 small melon
» 2 oranges

METHOD

1. Slice the carrots in half and feed them through the juicer. Peel and de-seed the melon, then juice. Mix well with the orange juice and pour into chilled glasses.

RUNNING BENEFITS

This fabulous mix of fruit and vegetables gives you an antioxidant-rich immune-system boost, providing vitamins A, C and E. It has plenty of potassium too, to support healthy blood pressure.

NUTRITIONAL INFORMATION (PER PERSON)

188 calories; 4.2g protein; 41.9g carbohydrate; 0.5g fat (0.3g polyunsaturated, 0g monounsaturated, 0.2g saturated); 7.82g fibre

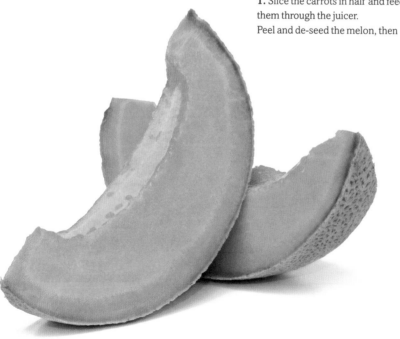

STRAWBERRY MILKSHAKE SMOOTHIE

REPLACE ENERGY POST-RUN WITH THIS SWEET, FRUITY DRINK

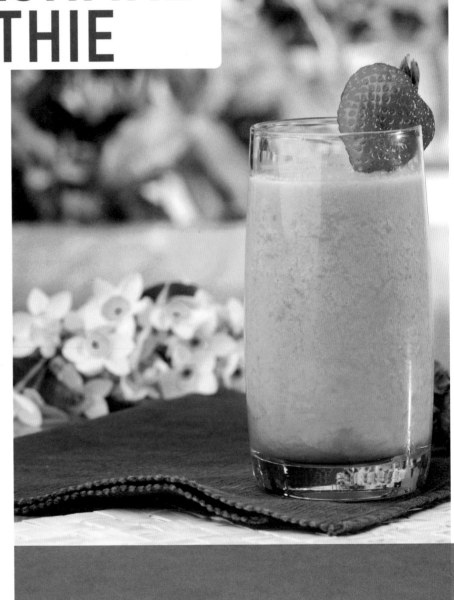

PREPARATION
Serves: 1
Preparation: 5 minutes

INGREDIENTS
▸▸ 400g strawberries
▸▸ 250ml skimmed milk
▸▸ Dash of honey

METHOD
1. Put the strawberries into a blender and blitz until smooth. Pour in the milk and blitz for a few more seconds. Then pour into a chilled glass and add a dash of honey.

RUNNING BENEFITS
This is a perfect post-run shake, providing a good mix of protein and carbohydrates for energy replenishment and muscle repair.

NUTRITIONAL INFORMATION (PER PERSON)
197 calories; 11.7g protein;
38.8g carbohydrate; 0.5g fat;
(0g polyunsaturated,
0.2g monounsaturated,
0.3g saturated); 4.4g fibre